MEDICINAL PLANTS

MEDICINAL PLANTS

Sunita Singh
Subhalaxmi

KALPAZ

ISBN: 978-81-7835-986-1

Price: ₹ 750

First Published 2013

Published by

Kalpaz Publications
C-30, Satyawati Nagar,
Delhi - 110052
E-mail: kalpaz@hotmail.com Ph.: 9212142040
Laser Typesetting : Rajender Vashist, Delhi
Printed at: G. Print Process, Delhi

Cataloging in Publication Data--DK
Courtesy: D.K. Agencies (P) Ltd. <docinfo@dkagencies.com>

Singh, Sunita.
Medicinal plants / Sunita Singh, Subhalaxmi.
p. cm.
Includes bibliographical references and index.
ISBN 9788178359861

1. Medicinal plants--India--Classification. 2. Botanical drug industry--India. 3. Consumer behavior--Environmental aspects--India.
I. Subhalaxmi, joint author. II. Title.

DDC 581.6340954 23

Contents

भारतीय लोक प्रशासन संस्थान
इन्द्रप्रस्थ एस्टेट, रिंग रोड, नई दिल्ली-110 002 स दूरभाष : 23702400 (15 लाइन)
INDIAN INSTITUTE OF PUBLIC ADMINISTRATION
INDRAPRASTHA ESTATE, RING ROAD, NEW DELHI-110002 (INDIA)

T.N. Chaturvedi
Chairman, IIPA
Former Governor of Karnataka
Former Member of Parliament (R.S.)
Former Comptroller & Auditor General of India

Tel : 011-23705927 (O)
011-23702400
95120-4214025 (R)

Foreword

India is very rich in Biodiversity, housing around 6-12% of total world's species of plants. This mega-diversity is intricately related to the socio-cultural practices of the country. The origin of 'Ayurveda' is from this region and first well documented use of herbal medicines is given by 'Acharya Dhanvantri' much before the origin of the western systems of medicine. In India, more than 80% people still depend on traditional systems of medicines and use herbal medicines because of their faith in the system and its easy access and affordability. This is also a well known fact that most of the medicines of Ayurveda, Unani, Homeopathy and Alopathy are directly and indirectly derived from the plants. We have over 2500 plant species in India, well documented for medicinal value. The Government of India has set up 'The National Biodiversity Authority in 2003 to implement the Biological Diversity Act 2002. I do hope an efforts like this by two dedicated and knowledgeable authors will help to promote research on the area.

The State of Jharkhand is rich in natural resources. Because of unique edaphic and climatic conditions, there are number of endemic plant species. Dr. Sumita Singh and Dr. Subhalaxmi book on 'Marketing Management of Medicinal and Aromatic plants of Jharkhand' is a remarkable compilation of types of plants and outlining the importance of plants of medicinal and aromatic significance. The seven chapters of the book provide knowledge of these plants as well as their marketing potential in India and abroad.

In developing countries, the most important thing is sustainable harvest of these plants and plant parts so that they are available for future generation.; the book will be extremely useful for the medical professionals, foresters, botanists, pharmacologists for its valuable information about plants as well as for business people to understand the marketing potential and gaps is marketing strategy for these plants with a view to maximize the potential for marketing.

I congratulate the authors for compilation of very useful storehouse of information, which is needed by common man to and fro business man in Jharkhand and other part of the country,. I wish that they can come out with similar information for other states as well. I wish Dr. Sumita Singh and her colleague Dr. Subhalaxmi all success in their imaginative and greatly needed mission.

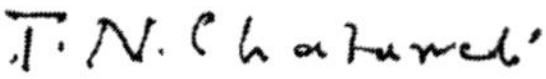

(T.N. Chaturvedi)

Preface

This book presents the international Marketing growth of Medicinal Plants. It represents a wide scope of plants especially herbal plants, India has rich diversity of medicinal plants, The supply base of 90 per cent herbal raw drugs used in the manufacture of Ayurveda, Siddha, Unani and Homoeopathy systems of medicine is largely from the wild. This wild source is speedily shrinking day-by-day due to deforestation. Therefore, there is a need for conservation and sustainable use of medicinal plants. Cultivation is clearly a sustainable alternative to the present collection of medicinal plants from the wild. This can be a potential provider of returns to the farmers. The work highlights the necessity of continued and integrated research on Marketing of Medicinal Plants in India, It also focuses on the need for proof of efficacy and safety in drug development and the need to recognise societies contributing plant materials.

The development of safe and effective medicinal and aromatic plant products depends upon the collaborative efforts of cultivators, collectors, conservationists, processors and businesses along with those of educators, sociologists, researchers and investors in developed and developing societies. This work shows the progress that can be made by further developing this collaboration to enhance the discovery, production and use of medicinal and aromatic plants.

Sunita Singh
Subhalaxmi

Introduction

The use of plants for preparations of medicines and in health care is by and large the largest use of plants in terms of the number of species specifically targeted. Plants provides the predominant ingredients of medicines used in most traditional systems of healing and also have been the source of inspiration for several major pharmaceutical drugs development. India is known for its various traditional system of medicines that have been developed and practised from time immemorial. A large number of traditional healing systems such as Ayurveda, Sidda, tribal medicines, folk medicines, etc., are widely practised for treatments of very complex and complicated diseases like cancers to simple requirement of primary health care. As per the WHO estimate about 80 per cent of the world population are depending greatly on these Traditional health care systems for their primary health care needs. Modern medicines are yet to be accessible to mass for various obvious reasons. The scale of trade in MAPs ranges from local to international. However, decision makers usually have little awareness of the significance of trade and consumption of medicinal plants, or of the problems of un-sustainability and sometimes harmful impacts on natural habitats of wild collection. Hence, much of the trade is unrecorded or poorly documented in official statistics.

Sunita Singh
Subhalaxmi

1

Need of Medicinal Plants

1.1 Need of Medicinal Plants

The use of plants as source of medicines and human sustenance has been in vogue since antiquity. India has a rich heritage of use of plants as medicines. Indian systems of medicines utilise 80 per cent of the material derived out of plants. There are over 2,500 plant species in India having documented medicinal value. 1Global estimates indicate that 80 per cent of population can not afford the products of western pharmaceutical industry and have to rely upon the use of traditional medicine mainly derived from plants. 2The literature on medicinal plants is quite vast, scattered and not available at one place. A great necessity was felt to have relevant Literature at one place providing multidisciplinary information on such resources. The research entitled. 'Marketing of medicinal plants in India with special reference to the state of Jharkhand will provide information on commercial plants available for trade and drug industry. It will facilitate to identify the essential oils, plants causing health hazards, having ethion medical importance and species suitable for incorporation in cropping systems in different climatic zones of India in general and the state of Jharkhand in particular. The research will serve as a useful companion to industrialists, collectors cultivators, foresters, planners, nature lovers, businessmen, those interested to know the details of Indian systems of medicines Ayurveda, unani, Homeopathy, Pharmacognosy and Ethnomedicines.

India has a rich heritage of use of plants as medicines, majority of them growing in a wild state like Jharkhand and Himachal Pradesh. Traditional systems of medicines continue to be widely practiced. According to a survey report by WHO, about 25 per cent of prescribed human medicines are derived from plants and 80 per cent people still depend on traditional systems of medicines[3].

Due to heavy demand from pharmaceutical industry leading to over exploitation, destruction of habitants and un sustainable harvesting practices suns conservation and cultivation support many valuable herbs especially in the Himalayan region are the state of Jharkhand are facing the danger to their survival in their natural abode. The knowledge of status of existing resources particularly their biosystematics and utilisation potential are the perquisites for conservation in its broad sense. Much is desired to formulate a comprehensive strategy to cover identification, Collection, Storage, preservation, sustainable utilisations, supply, restoration of the ecological balance and regeneration aspects. An insight into ethnobotanical aspects provides an added fillip to the efforts, unraveling the natures mysterious and miraculous generosities. This grass root approach to local inventory will enrich and strengthen. The macro approach of national and global biodiversity enumerations. Important plants include the name, description, distribution in the different parts of India in general and state of Jharkhand in particular, parts used, chemical constitutes medical uses, MARKET PRICES, cultivation notes supported by data on COMMERCIAL IMPORTANCE, BUSINESS POTENTIAL, listing of ended danger species scope for PHARMACEUTICAL INDUSTRIES, scope of cultivation is different agroclimatic zones. Potential substitutes formulation in Indian systems of medicines.

Medicinal plants play an important role in human life to combate disease since time immemorial. The rural folks and tribal in India in general and the state of Jharkhand in particular even new depend Largely on the surrounding plants / forests for their day to day needs. Medicinal plants are being looked upon not only on a source of health care but also as a SOURCE OF INCOME, The medicinal plants sector can provide a huge EXPORT OPPORTUNITY after fulfilling domestic needs. There is a NEED TO MAKE A RESEARCH with a view to promote integrated development by co-ordinating. Stimulating production, processing MARKETING and establishing a sound infrastructure to the medicinal plant sector in India in general and the state of Jharkhand in particular. Our study aims to make an in-depth study of MARKET POTENTIAL of medicinal plants and its sustainable management a people movement in India in general and the state of Jharkhand in particular.

The varied agro climate conditions in the country like India and the state of Jharkhand make it suitable for growing a wide range and variety of medicinal plants. The production of medicinal plants being labour intensive generates increased employment opportunities for the farmers particularly the rural masses of India and tribals of the state of Jharkhand and enhances their income. Growing medicinal plants is much more remunerative as compared to growing cereals horticultural crops etc., both in India and the state of Jharkhand. The value of medicinal plants related trade in India is of the order of 5.5 billion U.S. dollar (Exium Bank Report 1997) and in further increasing day-by-day. The international market of herbs product is estimated to be US$ 62 billion. India's share in the global market of medicinal plants trade is less than 0.5 per cent. In view of the innate India strengths, which includes diverse eco-systems for growth of medicinal plants, technical farming capacity, strong manufacturing sector, the medicinal plants, technical forming capacity, strong manufacturing sector, the medicinal plants sector can provide EXPORT OPPORTUNITY after fulfilling domestic needs.

The Indian systems of medicines suffer from the confusion and controversies due to prevalent synonyms. Many names are assigned to a plant species and the same name is applicable to many different species. To facilitate the physician and the pharmaceutical expert in selecting, the genuine drug, there is a prime need to minimise, if not the altogether removal of controversies and confusion by identifying the genuine material adulterants and substitutes and establishing standard and that could he adopted uniformly throughout the country. Hence, researches in herbal drugs and more so, the process of discovering new and valuable drugs from plants, brings together various discipline like Taxonomy, Pharmacognosy, Phytochemistry, Pharmacology, Toxicology and Clinical screening.

Keeping in view the recent, growing popularity of herbal remedies. The Indian medicinal plants, more so the Himalyan herbs have received in unpresented attention world, over. The literature on medicinal plants in quite vast, scattered and not available at one place even in big libraries. A great necessity was felt to haves relevant literature providing multi disciplinary information on such resources. The present resource work will serve the cause of the readers from diverse categories who have the curiosities to know the plants and make use of them.

1.2. Medicinal Plants : A Conceptual Approach

Herbal medicine include herbs, herbal materials, herbal preparations and finished herbal products that contain as active ingredents parts of plants, or other plant materials, or combinations. Traditional use of herbal medicines refers to the long historical use of these medicines. Their use is well established and widely acknowledged to be safe and effective, and may be accepted by national authorities.[4]

The World Health organisation (WHO) has defined herbal medicines as finished labelled medicinal products that contain as active ingredients aerial or under ground parts of plants or other plant material or combination there on whether in the crude state or as plant preparations. The same WHO document adds that medicines containing plant material combined with chemically defined active substances, including chemically defined, isolated constituents of plants, are not considered to be herbal medicines. The goal of health for all can not be achieved without herbal medicines.

Herbal medicinal, as defined by WHO, can be classified into three categories.

1. Phytomedicines or photo phytopharmaceuticals sold as over the counter (OTC) products in modern dosage forms as tablets capsules and liquids for oral use.
2. Dietary supplements containing herbal products, also called nutraceuticals available in modern dosage forms.

   These two types of herbal medicines are used by consumers in developed countries and those in urban areas of developing countries. These herbal medicines are gradually occupying increasing shelve space in modern pharmacies.
3. Herbal medicines consisting of either crude, semi-processed or processed medicinal plants. These have a vital place is primary health care in developing countries.

In order to have a clear concept of medicinal plants the under noted terms pertaining to it must be taken into consideration.

2.1 The Antiquity Herbal Medicine[5]

The earliest recorded evidence of their use in Indian, Chinese, Greek, Roman and Syrian texts dates back to about 5,000 years. The classical Indian texts include RIGVEDA, ATHARVA VEDA, CHARAKA SAMHITA and SUSHRUTA SAMHITA. The herbal medicines traditional medicines have therefore been derived from rich traditions or ancient civilisations and scientific heritage and had come to the present generations through oral traditions. Ancient literature me also mentions herbal medicines for age related diseases namely memory loss osteoporosis, diabetic wounds, immune and Liver disorders etc. for which modern medicine or only palliative therapy is available.

2.2 Nutraceuticals[6]

This is a term of recent origin (1979) and comprises simple terms. It is nothing but nutritionally or medicinally enhanced foods. These include engineered gain cereals supplemented with vitamins or minerals, or genetically manipulated osylean and canola oil without transfalty acids. Many pharma and biotech companies have moved into this area since it does not involve regulatory clearance and offer large markets.

Nutraceuticals are in great demand in the developed world particularly USA and Japan. Nutraceutical market in U.S.A alone is about $ 80-250 billion, with a similar market size in Europe and Japanese sales worth $ 1.5 billion. Such huge markets have arisen because of the Dietary supplement Health Education Act passed by U.S.A. in 1994, which permits unprecedented claims to bee made about food or the dietary supplement's ability about health benefits including prevention and treatment of diseases. In 1996, the U.S. Herbal medicine market was about $ 4 billions and with the current growth rate may be more than double by the turn of the century. Amongst the developed countries Germany holds the lead and has published individual monograph on therapeutic benefits of more than 300 herbs. In developing countries China has compiled generated data an over 800 medicinal plants and exports large Quantities of herbal drugs. India has prepared only few monographs and its exports are dismal.

2.3. Herbal Medicine Standardisation[7]

Medicinal plant parts should be anthentic and free from harmful materials like pesticides, heavy metals, microtia or radioactive contamination, etc. The extract should then be checked foindicated biological activity in an experimental animal model(s). The bio-active extract should be standardised on the basic of active principal or major compound(s) along with fingerprints The next important step in stabilisation of the bioactive extract with a minimum shelf of over year.

2.4 Value Added Products[8]

The raw materials used in the herbal preparations must be used for :

(1) Isolation of active ingredients for formulation into drugs.

(2) IsoLation of intermediates for the production of semisynthetic drugs.

(3) Preparation of standardised galenicals (extracts powder, tinctures etc.)

3. Quality Assurance[9]

The control of the Quality of the raw materials, finished products and processes is an absolute necessity to complete in the international market. The production of traditional medicines for local use does not require such stringent standards.

India is sitting on a gold mine of well recorded and well practiced knowledge of traditional herbal medicine. But unlike China, India has not been able to acpitalise on this herbal wealth by promoting its use in the developed world despite their renewed interest in herbal medicines. This can be achieved by judicious product identifications based on diseases found in the developed world for which no medicine or only palliative therapy is available; such herbal medicines will find speedy access into those countries.

3.1 Herbal Medicine Scenario in India[10]

The turnover of herbal medicines in India over the counter products, ethical and classical formulations and home remedies of AYURVEDA, UNANI and SIDHA system of medicines is about a billion dollar with a meager export of about $80 billion.

Three of the 10 most widely selling herbal medicines in the developed countries, namely preparations of Allium sativalim Aloe barbedensis and panax species are available in India.

About 1500 Plants with medicinal uses are mentioned in ancient texts and around 800 plants have been used in traditional medicine with or without standardisation. In 1989 WTO developed were ratified by the 6th International conference of Drug Regulatory Authorities held at ottawa. The salient features of W.H.O guidelines are :

(1) Quality assess ment crude plant material, plant preparation; finished product.

(2) Stability shelf life.

(3) Safety assessment Documentation safety based on experience or/and Toxicology studies.

(4) Assessment of efficacy: Documented evidence of traditional use or/and activity determination (animals, human).

3.2 Tribal System of Treatment[11]

The tribal society has largely depended upon its traditional knowledge about tribal medicine, mainly based on medicinal herbs commonly found in the area for treatment of disease generally prevalent in the area and for melting contingencies such as snake and insect bites.

Tribal system of treatment is a strange mixture of magic and medicine, of faith in super natural elements and in medicinal herbs. With spread of education and literacy and with greater facilities for availing modern medical treatment, the belief that diseases are caused by hostile spirit angered by violation of some taboos I does no longer have that dominate hold on the tribal mind that it used to have in the past. But this is not true of their faith in curative properties of herbs which is still unshaken. The first choice of tribal people is if the herbs are available and the medicine man is around, to get them selves treated in the indigenous way.

It was found that the most common diseases were malaria, cold and coguh, fever, typhoid, diahrroea and dysentery. Diseases related to abdominal joyriders like diahrroea and dysentery are also very common. The sufferings from these in most cases continued up to one week. By and large, in treatment of most common diseases predominantly allopathic medicines were used followed by herbal medicines.

One of the important reason for prevalence of intestinal diseases in remote rural areas is the lack of safe drinking water. The situation is likely to improve with the installation of hand pumps. But where this facility is not available, people have to be depend upon unsake, unhygenic sources like river water wells, darichas and nallahs and therefore incidence of such disorders is high. Diseases caused by malnurition such as anaemia and night blindness are also common. So also are cases of liver disorders such as jaundice, perhaps, caused by addition to drinks.

4.1 Sources of Knowledge About Herbal Medicines[12]

In the tribal area of chhotanagpus out of the total 913 households, 765 i.e. 83.79% of the households did not have their own knowledge about herbal medicines. Among 149 i.e. 16.32% households possessing knowledge of herbal medicine, The sources of such knowledge were identified as parents, relatives, friends and other. In many households there were multiple source of knowledge. The main source of the information about herbal medicines were relatives (62, 56%). Thus in these households the source of knowledge about herbal medicine was by the large, limited to a small circle of family, friends and kingships groups. The majority of the households i.e. 83.79% were totally dependent upon tribal medicine men and other outside sources.

(i) Procurement of Herbal Medicine in the Tribal Area of Chhota Nagpur[13]

In the tribal areas of chhota nagpur there are two main sources for procurement of herbal medicines. These were OJHA/BAITH and forest. When a tribal family consuets a practitioner is herbal medicines it gets the supply of necessary herbs from him or in same cases he is helped to identify the herbs and asked to get it from the nearly forest.

References

1. Plant Breeders and Farmers in the New Intellectual Property Regime: Conflict of Interests (J.F. Science Publishers Inc, New Hampshire p. 177.
2. Gadgil, M and Devasia, P., 1995, Intellectual Property Rights and Biological Resources : Specifying geographical origins and prior knowledge of uses, pp. 637-39.
3. P. Ganguli, 1998, Gearing for Patents : The Indian Scenario, University press, Hyderabad.
4. Prakam, S. 1999, Shantharam S. Montgomery, The I.P.R. Debate in India in Biotechnology Biosafety and Biodiversity, J.F. Science Publishers. Inc, New Hampshire, pp. 225-226.
5. Shanthgram, S., and Montgomery (eds.), The I.P.R controversy and the Indian Seed Industry (In Biotechnology, Biosafety, and Biodiversity, J.F. Science Publishers, Inc, New Hampshire, pp. 225-226.
6. Shanthgram, S, and Montgomery (eds), The IPR controversy and the Indian seed Industry (In Biotechnology, Biosqfety and Biodiversity, J.F. Science Publishers, Inc., New Hampshine, pp. 207-218.
7. Swaminathan M.S. 1993, A Plant Variety Protection for India.
8. The Encyclopedic Source Texts of Ayurvede. (Samhithas).
9. Charaka Samhita (Commentary of Chakrapani), Acharyay. T. Nirnayasagar Press, Bombay, 1941.
10. Aggarwal, V.S. and Ghosh, B. Drug plants of India (Root Drugs Kalyani Publishers, New Delhi 1985.

11. Medicinal Plants of India. Vol. I, Anonymous, I.C.M.R. New Delhi 1976.
12. The Ayurvedic Formulary of India Part-I, Anonymous, Government of India New Delhi 1978.
13. Dravya Vignana Shastra, Ashwatha Harayan, Ayurveda Mahavidalaya Maysore 1960.

Further Reading

Bailey, L.H., Manual of Cultivatied plants, The Macmillan.

Boericke, W., Pocket Manual of Homeopathic, Material Medica, Jain Publishers, New Delhi 1991.

Chopra, R.N., Chopra, I.C, Handa, K.L.C. and Kapur, L.D., Chopra's India enous Drugs of India 2nd., Academic Publishers Calcutta 1958-1994.

Chopra, R.N., Nayar. S.L. and Chopra I.C., *Glossary of Indian Medicinal Plants.*

CSIR, New Delhi 1956.

Bhavaprakasha

Nighantu (Indian Material Medica)

Sri Bhavamisra, Chaukambna

Bharti Academy, Vaaranasi-1984

2

Types of Medicinal Plants in India

Demand for Medicinal Plants, across the globe is increasing. The world Health Organisation has estimated that 80 per cent of the population of the developing countries rely on herbal medicines even in the developed countries the market for herbal medicines is growing faster than that for other pharmaceutical products.

However, the supply of medicinal plants today is not adequate to meet the world herbal demand which is currently growing at a rate of seventy per cent per annum. Currently. Bulk of the medicinal plant, material is being collected from the wild. It is estimated that 95 per cent of medicinal plants collected in India is gathered from the wild.[1]

In India Medicinal Plants are also numerous. It is estimated that some 10,000 plant species are used medicinally.[2]

In India alone, over 7,500 species of plants are estimated to the used by the ethnic comminutes.[3]

The Andhra Pradesh's principal chief conservation of Forests, Mr. S.D. Mukherji, said currently the Indian system of medicine such as Ayurveda Unani and Siddha used over 1,100 medicinal plants most of them collected from the wild. About one lakh medical manuscripts are available in oriental libraries and private collections in India and abroad, but only a few hundred of these books are said to be available to the students and teachers of Indian medicine.

According to Dr. S. Vedavathy, President of the Herbal Folk lore.

Research Centre at Tirupati, these are several reasons for the medicinal plants not being cultivated one of them is the low cost of wild material besides, a cultivated material requires agricultural expertise time, Land and financial resources among other things. Another factor is the dearth of knowledge on the identity and ago-technology of the plants needed.[4]

The National Bank for Agriculture and Rural Development (NABARD) has prepared general guidelines so as to help other Banks to formulate schemes for the development of medicinal plants. It has also provided models on the cost of development of medicinal plants such as Rauvolfa Serpentine and Atropa Belladonna.[5]

But, so far, the achievement under this sector is insignificant, still there is no adequate information on suitable areas of cultivation, economic size of the unit, gestation period of the plant, parts used harvesting procedures post - harvest handling intermediate processing procedures, packing and storage requirements.[6]

India represents one of the eight important centres of origin and crop plant diversity of cultivated plants and their wild relatives. It is immensely rich in medicinal and aromatic plants occurring in diverse eco-systems. World Health Organisation (WHO) has listed over 21,000 plant species used around the world for medicinal purposes (National Bureau of Plant Genetic Resources, NBPGR booklet 1996. It has been estimated that India has, 47000 species of plants and is no 8 in world biodiversity out of these medicinal plants compress of 8,000 species. Indian system of Medicine (ISM) uses around 2,500 plants species belonging to more than 1000 genera. About 800 species are used by industry of which approximately 25 per cent are cultivated.[7]

The descriptive profile of Medicinal and Achromatic Plants of India are as under:

ABIES SPECTABILIS (D.DON) SPACH[8]

Description : A lofty tree of great height leaves flattered, linerav, 2.5 - 7.5 cm, spirally arranged around the branches, tip notched, upper surface dark green, shining, lower with a silvery white line on each side of the midrib with incurved margins.

Parts Used : Leaves

Current Market Rate : Rs. 6 to Rs. 10 per kg for dried needles in local markets.

Distribution : Afghanistan to Bhutan, 2800 - 4000 m spreading over large areas in the upper tree zone. Common in Himachal

Pradesh between 3600 - 4200 m forming climatic climax and often goes upto 4500 m.

Local/Common Name(s) : Himalayan High - Level Silver-Fir, Kolroi, Tosh, Talispatra.

Flowering / Fruiting: April - May, cones ripen during September - October.

Properties and uses : The leaves in the form of decoction or infusion are anusedin chronic bronchitis, phthsis and other pulmonary affections. It is also reported as antiflatulent, antispasmodic, appetiser, astringent, earminative digestive, diwretic, expectorant, feverlfuge stomachic and tonic. It is considered poisonous in large doses powdered leaves alongwith juice of Justice Ahatoda (*Vasaka*) and honey are used in hemoptsis, phthisis and in catarrah of bladder. Infusion of leaves is given to infants suffering from fever and chest infection; also in hoarseness and during dentition. In Ayurveda, the plant is also mentioned as contraceptive, leaf Juice is antiperiodic. The name talispatra given to it is still controversial. In many parts of the country it is used, whereas in others Taxus Wallichiana Leaves are valued as tails and still in some parts Rhododen Dron Anthopogon Leaves are used as (Broad-Leaved talispatra) in indigenous preparations.

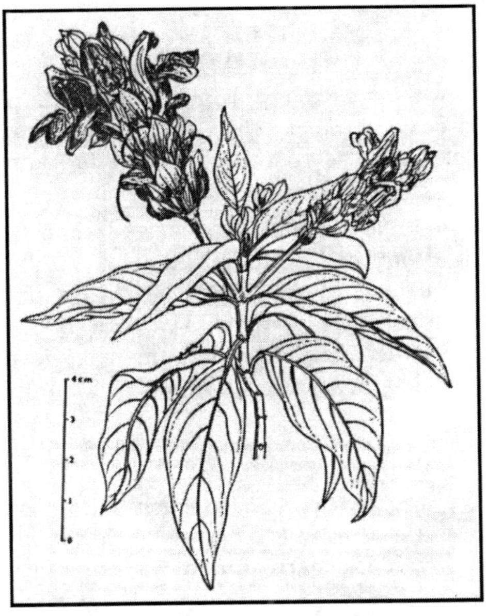

Fig. 1. Vasaka (Adhatoda Zeylanica).

(a) Talisadichurna
(b) Talisadivat
(c) Sudarshan Chunna
(d) Lavanbhash Churna
(e) Kanakasava

Cultivation

Propagation is through seeds. The percentage of fertile seeds produced by firs is much smaller than that yielded by spruce and pines. Seeds can not be safely stored for more than 1-2 years. Seeds are raised in carefully prepared nursery beds or polythene bags covered to a depth equal to the thickness of seeds in the soil. Seedlings are sensitive to heat of the sun and need protection by using bush screens. It can also be propagated by side grafting.

FAMILY

II. ABRUS PRECATORIUS LINN[9]

Description : A much branched climber with a woody stem. Leaves are paripinnate, 5-7.5 cm long leaflets 20-40, opposite, deciduous, oblong ligulate, membranous glabrous or thinly silky heneath. Flowers are reddish or white. calyx, campanulate, thinly silky, corollaovate, wing narrow, keen larger that wings, stamens qunited in sheath. Ovary many valued style small, pods oblong, 3 to 5 seeded, seeds ovoid or sub - globose, generally two third scarlet or white and the rest get black giving appearance of a black eye.

Parts Used : Roots is often known as Indian Liquorice. It is found in pieces of varying lengths, which are generally more oraless twisted and branched covered by a very thin pale browen or somewhat eddish benic. This surrounds a yellowish, woody portion, the fracture of which is short and somewhat feverous. It has sweetish and mucilaginous taste resembling with ordinary liquorice roots.

Use

(A) Seeds : Purgative, emetic tonic aphrodisiac, used is nervous disorders and cattle posioning. The seeds which are of a brilliant scarlet colour with black mark on one side are much employed as beads. In the past, jewellers made use of these seeds as a unit of measurement for weighing gold as "Ratti" young girls used to string these into necklaces and also for decoration of baskets, bracelets and rosaries.

(B) Poultice of Seeds : Used as suppository to bring aborion.

(C) Root : Emetic, all exiteric and the alcoholic extract of the seed kernels has analgesic and central nervous system depressant activity. The drug has spasmogenic effect and was bound to have relaxant effect on rat uterus (cadres 1986).

Main Ingredients: Seeds contain principal poisonous constituent abrin, a toxaemil similar to ricin from cast or seeds, a glucoside abrine alkaloldabashime. Roots and leaves contains precool, abroad and two alkaloid abraine and percussion.

Aqueous alcoholic extract yielded oriention and orientine (chobraetal 1956 and CCRAS 1986)

Preparations : Gunjadi taila, Gunja-pralepa etc.

Cultivation Notes : Can be cultivated through seeds sours in April - May. Seeds are soaked in water for 24 hours before being sown in the nursery can be sown directly in well spaced pits. It can also be propagated through slips. Since it is a dedicated climber, it requires support for its better performance. Either, temporary support has to be provided or it should be grown along fences and shrubberies. It can also be propagated by cuttings of firm shoots is sand under glass.

Flowering / Fruiting : September to January.

Local / Common names(s) : Ratti, Gunja, Chunti, Indian Liquorice, Crabs eye, Red bead vine, Prayer beads.

Family : Leguninosae.

ACACIA CATECHIS WILLD[10]

Family : Leguminosae

Local/ Common Name(s)

(a) Khair

Description : Acatechu is a moderate sized tree attaining a height of 1- to 13 m. In favourable localities, it attains a cylindrical stemup to 1.5 m is girth with 6 m hole. Ordinarily; it is a small tree with 60 - 90 cm girth and 2.4 - 3 m hole. Its greyish hroun bark is nearly 1.25 cm. is thickness, exboliating is long, narrow strips, brown or red inside. Branches are unarmed, Leaves are hipinnate, armed with stipulary. Thorns, occasionally having numerous leaflets. Flowers are small. White or pale yellow in axillary spikes (1- 4 together). Corolla 5 cleft, petal united, stamens distinct, pods thin, flat, glabrous, 4-8 seeded.

Flowering/ Fruiting: May - June to October.

Parts Used : Heart wood, extract (katha). The sapwool is thick red, turning, brownish red to realy blank with age.

Current Market Rate : Khair hark Rs. 10 per kg. katha Rs. 190 to 370 per kg.

Main ingredients : Contains catechin, catechutanic acid and tannin wood contains ox (Alfha) B (Beta) and Y (Gamma) catechien, and 1- epicatechin.

Uses : The cutch obtained from the heatwood of over 20-30 yrs old trees is used as important ingredient of paan. Chewed extensively in India. It is a useful raw material for ply wood adhesives and is extensively used for dyeing canvas, fishing nets and ropes.

Various plant parts are used in sord-mouth chest plain, cancer, colic pain, gravel, pthisis, bronchial asthma, consumption and strangulation of intestine, Bak juice alongwith asafoetida is used in hemoptysis. Important drug for leprosy in Ayurveda.

Bark is used as astringent, digestive and useful for cough and diarrhoea. It is useful in rbronchilaffections, cancer, piles, sorethroat, ulceration obstinate skin diseases including different forms of leprosy. Gum from the dark is considered a good substitute for gum arabic. The tree observes as a host for lac insect "Kheerbal", a product met with is some older tree in the form of white crystalline deposit of catechin is used for the treatment of cough and sone throat. Mixture of flower tops, cuminsis given is gonorrhoea.

Preparation

1. Khadirad; Vat,
2. Khadirarishta,
3. Khadir - sar,
4. Lavangadi - Vati,
5. Chandanadi - Vati,
6. Kutafarista etc.

Cultivation Notes : Seeds can be collected during December to January and sown in February to March is polythene bag of nursery - beads. Before sowing, the seeds should be immersed in water for 24 hours seedlings are ready for transplanting after 6 months. Direct sowing of the seed is successful for gapply orestation astrans planting can not be relied upon, because of its fragile root system. Soaking of seeds in cold water for 24 hours gives good germination. The tree can also be propagated through root and shoot cuttings (stumps) made from seedlings of about 15 months old. Planting of stumps should be done soon after the break of rains. Sowing Khair seed is lines alongwith the agricultural crops acts as the cheapest and the best method. The seeds and young plants demand plenty of light, moisture lack of weeds and should be planted at a spacing of 2.5 × 2.5 m to 3 × 3 m. where conditions are favourable. They grow to a height of 1.5 to 1.8 m within a year. Two regular thinnings up to the age of about ten years are required and are repeated at intervals of five to six years.

ACACIA NILOTICA DELIFE. SUPP. INDICA (BENTH) BRENAN SYN. A ARBICAWILLD[11]

Family : Leguminosae

Local/Common Name(s)

(i) Kikar,

(ii) Babul.

Flowering/ Fruiting : July - Sep to April to June :

Description : A moderate sized tree with large spreading crown, bark drawbar almost black much fissured, spines 1,25.0, cm long straight white sharply pointed, leaves 2.5 - 5.0 cm long, rachis and pinnae downy pinnate 3-6 pairs, 1.25 to 3.0 cm long with several glands at their insertions, leaflets 10-20 pairs, 0.25 to 0.50 cm long, liners, glabrous. Flowers yellow, fragrant in axillary, globose heads which are about 1.25 cm diameter, pedicles is fascicles of 3-5, short slender, greydowny, with a short of bracts above the middle, calyx cup-shaped, 0.1 cm long corolla twice the length of ealyx. Pod generally solitary, 4- 6 by 1.25 - 1.50 cm, 8.12 seeded, stalked convex, rather, fleshy deeply indented between the seeds, densely grey-downy, tardily dehiscent.

Parts Used : Heart wood, Gum, Pod, Bark

Current - Market Rate : Bark Rs. 8-10 per kg.

Properties and uses : Heart wood is used for wheels, well-C urbs, sugar and oil presses, rice powders and for ploughs and other agricultural implements. Gum is used in sore throat. Alongwith latex of calotropisprocera, It is given to cure asthma, stops bleeding urinary and vaginal dischanges and is also useful is diabetes. Bark is cooling and anthill mintic. It cures skin diseases, bleeding piles etc. Bark is also used as substitute for soap. The pod is a favorite food for cattle sheep and goats, used in impotency and effective in urinogenital disorders. It is also very much in tannin before ripening. Flowers cause allergy. flowers pods and gum resins are used as tonic in diarrhoea and dysentery. Bruised leaves are applied to sore eyes in children, eaten in throat infection and popultice is used in sore eyes. Paste of the burnt leaves in effective ointment in itch. Various plant. Plants are used against hairfall, earach, syphilis, cholera, dysentrery, leprosy, and rinderpest. Ethye alchol (50%) extract of bark is antiprotozoal, hypotensive and spasmolytic.

Preparations

1. Babul, Aristaand and lavangadi, bati.
2. Babul Tooth Paste.
3. Cultivation Notes.

Can be raised through seeds - seedlings can be planted as road side avenue wind breaks and shelter belts aswellas biofence in field of baunders.

ACHILLEA MILLE FOLIUM LINN[12]

Family : Composite

(Asteraceae)

Local/Common Name(s)

1. Birnjasib

Flowering/Fruiting : July - September

Description : A small peremmial tufted herb upto 50 cm tall, with a slender cropping root stock, throwing numerous roots and stolns with blunt succulent scale at each node. Leaves alternate, along - lanceolate, 3- pinnatisect, minutely divided into linear, dentate, mucromate more or less hairy segments. Flowers are numerous, small, white in corymbose ovoid flat topped heads at the ends of stems and branches fruit shining.

Parts Used : *Leaves and flower heads/ entire plant*

Properties and uses : It has been used from early times for a great variety of medicinal purposes and has been given as infusion or liquid extract. It is stated to have diurectic, strimulant and haemostatic properties in the dose of 2-4 gm (mrtiudale, 1977). In many parts of Europe, a decoction of the leaves and flower heads is employed as a carminatives tonic and aromatic, stimulating (Dec. 1980). Due to the presence of choline it has hypotensive effect, (chopraetal - 1969). The leaves and flower heads are also used as a tonic and vapour bath for fever. The herb is employed as a substitute for hope in some parts of Sweden is the preparation of bles and is thought to render it more intoxicating. Its not infusion is used as an emmenagogue in France (watt 1972). Yarrow tea is good remedy for sever colds, fevers and obstructed per aspiration. A decoction of the whole plant is employed for bleeding piles and is good for kidney diseases, also prevents boldness (Grieve, 1959) Medicated vapour both containing yarrow, Lavender flowers wheat brain and milk is used in nasal catrrh and fever. It has a specific action on the pelvic organs and is used is amenorrhoea, menorrhagia and leucorrhoea. As a hilter tonic, it is given during convalescence from fevers and is atomic dyspepsia to promote appetite. Its chief use is relaxation of sprinter and with discharge of mucus or blood during defecation. The inbusion is applied to relax throat and sore nipple with benefits (Khoty and katsak, 1984) local inhalitante chew the leaves to relieve tooth - ache as it produces a pungent but - tingling and cooling sensations bringing immediate relief.

Preparations : Liv. 52, livergen, livomyn etc.

Cultivation Notes: Propagated by divisions of roots and through seeds. Since the plant produces a number of suckers, these can be separated and transplanted in the field at a spacing of 30 cm × 30 cm during spring. It produces profuse quantity of seeds and can also be grown through seeds sown in nurseries and trems planted during pre-monsoons is the field having loamy, humus rich soils. It thrives and smaller spaces around and fields. Seed sown plants bear flowers in the second year.

ACHYRANTHES ASPERA LINN[13]

Family : AMARANTHACEAE Local/Comman Name (s)

(i) Puthkanda

Description : An erect herb about 0.5.2 m high with often a woody rootstock and much branched, acute out use or acuminate 4-10 cm × 2-5 cm, sparingly hairy with a short petiole. I Lowers are qrcen or pinkish crowded is 2-4 cm terminal spikes which elongate in fruit and reach up to 50 cm is length with young and upper flowers ascending and order and lower flower descending flat against the stem. Perianth glalerous and shining, stamens 5, alternating with truncate, staminodes. Fruit is an along utricle enclosed is the hardened perianth.

Flowering/Fruiting : April - September.

Parts used : whole plants.

Mainingredients : From the seeds, two saponins saponin A and saponin B have been isolated, saponin a methy, ester, B - methy/ester, have also been found. Alcoholic extract of the root yielded saponins. Saponins from the seed have cardiotonic activity. Saponins possess anti inflammatory activity besides potentiating the inhibitory response to the adrenal line (CRAS, 1990).

Preparations

(i) Aqastya-haritaki,

(ii) Kaphaketu - rasa,

(iii) Apamarga Kshara.

Used : The seeds are given in hydropholia in cases of snake bite, in ophthalmia and cutaneous diseases. The flowering spikes rubhed with a little sugar are made into pills and given internally to patients bitten by mad dogs. The pulp of fresh leaves applied externally is a good remedy for scorpion stings. The ash of the plant mixed with conjee is a remedy in dropsy. Saponins outained from the seeds have cardiotonic and diuretic activity. Saponins from the plant have been reported to possess anti-inflammatory activity besides potenting the inphibitory response to the adrenaline. Solvent extract of the aerial parts saved contraceptive and hormonal properties in rat (of CCRAS, 1990:16). Root is used as an abortifacient in local folklores and the kheer prepared of its seeds allays appetile and one does not require food for a couple of day on having its kheer.

Cnetivation noles : It is a very hardy plant and can grow in any type of conditions up to 1500 m elevation. Propagation is through seeds which can be broadcast is the field or souren is lines at a spacing of 45 × 45 cm during March-April. It is growth has been found quite luxuriant even without much of the inputs at Nauni (1250 m). Harvesting of erial shoots is done at full fruiting state. Root stock, being perennial throws out vigorous shoots is the growing season.

Ahhlied Species : Achyran these bidentata Blume.

ACONITUM DEINO RRHIZUM STAPE FAMILY[14]

Family : RANUNCULACEAE

Local Common Name(s)

(i) Mohro,

Description : A tall, glabrous, biennial herb with paired tuberous roots. The daughter tubbers are conical rather alongate up to 15 cm long and 3.5 cm in diameter at the crown with few root fibres. The surface is dark brown and coarsely wrinkled Mother tubers are similar, but have longer filiform root fillers. The drug is very hard and horny and its starch is gelatinised during drying. Leaves are scattered reniform or ovate reniform, 5 - 10 cm long acute or obtuse, 5 pedatipartite alimost to the hase. Cauline leaves, sharbly toothed, lowest long petioled; flowers more than 2.5 cm long, bright blue to greenish blue with purple veines in terminal racemes which go up to 45 cm long. Fruit is a capsule hear bearing numerous seeds.

Flowering-Fruiting : July-September.

Parts used : Dried conical daughter tubes. The roots of A. chasmanthum and A. balfouri are also sold as vastsanabh. Since A. chasmanthum contains pseudoaconitine is large propertions, its use is medicines requires careful purification.

Current Market Rate : Rs. 70-110 per kg.

Used : Together with A balfori, it is the principal constituent of A. Ferox and is imported into England. It is a poisons and effect affects both the heart and central nervous system. In case of extreme toxicity, the heart stops and respiration is depressed with large doses, death is almost instantaneous, resulting in paralysis of heart or the respiratory centre with moderate toxic doses, there is a tingling of the tongue, mouth, stomach, skin followed by numbers anaesthesia, nausea, vomiting, diarrhoea, excessive salivation, weak and irregular pulse, difficult respiration and mass calor weakness may result. Externally, it is used with mustard oil as massage is neuralaia, paralysis and muscular rheumatism. Its application should be avoided in wonder or abrased skin as it may get absorbed and cause poisoning (chauhan, 1984. 98-99). Locally much used for removing body pains, but carefully. Root is smoked is toothache and body pains Leaves are employed to improve the flavour of country liceuor, Also used is leprosy, cholera, rheumatism, as tonic is diarrhoea and cough (Mahandhav, 1980).

Preparations

(i) Aanitundivati,

(ii) Laghu-vishgarbha taila.

(iii) Swalp-kasturi-bhairavrasa,

(iv) Sanjivanivati,

(v) Kaphketu-rasa etc.

Cultivation Notes : At present entire accurate supply is obtained from wild sources more so from horror Forest Division. In order to obtain drugs of standard quality, a more careful collection and cultivation of this herb is required. It is endemic is distribution is erstwhile Bushahar state (parts of Rohru, Rampur and Kinnaur). Its collection, marketing and export has also been barned being an endangered species.

Propagation is effected easily by division of roots either in late autumn or early spring. It prefers rich humus and deep loamy soil with partial shade can be propagated through seed and splits of root with collar having vegetative buds is the areas situated between 2500-3200 m ele - vation in forest margins. Seeds should be souer in spring is small seed heds and are transplanted when they are 5 cm tall. Harvesting/collection from the wild sources is done during autumn and calls for precaution and expertise to avoid poisoning incidents. Roots should be kept at a safer place away from the knowledge of children, women and ignorant persous till its disposal.

ACONITUM HETER OPHYLLUM WALL.[15]

Family : RANUNCULACEAE

Local Common Name(s)

(i) Atvisha

Description : An erect, Leafy herb having biennial paired, tuberous roots. Steps up to 1 m tall with broad, ovate or orlcic ular cordate, labed and toothed, shortly stalked or sesile, amplexicaule leaves. Lower leaves are long petioled, while the cauuline leaves are sessile, amplexicaule. Flowers bright-blue to yellow qreenish blue with purple veins in long, many flowered peduncles. Seeds are dark brown.

Flowering/Fruiting : July-September, seeds can be collected during September-October.

Currecct Market rate : Rs. 1300-2200 per kg.

Cuetivation Notes : Can be cultivated/propagated through seeds and by divisions: Flourishes well in humus rich soic, retentive of moisture, is sun or partial shade. It thrives best is places which have been used as halting bases for flocks of sheep and goats in temperate and sub-alpine pastures and is the fields, rich is organic matter, partially shady and sligntly moisture retentive. Seeds have to be shown during March-April after snow meets and the seedlings are trams planted at a distance of about 30 cm. is well prepared fields after to 2 months. Roots are collected during september-November from the wild and the some season is the third year from cuetivation. Roots are dried, freed from dust, root filires and graded before being of locked and stored.

ACORUS CALAM US LINN.[16]

Family : ARACEAF

Local Common Name(s)

(i) Bare

Flowering/Fruiting : April-August

Parts used : Cut and dried pieces of the aromatic rhizomes, which are generally flattened, Somewhat curved pieces, usually some inches in length and from about 1.2 cm to 2.5 cm is diameter. Externally, it has yellowish brown or fawn colour and is more or less shrunken and wrinkled; marked on its upper surface with the scars and fibrous vestiges of the leaves and on its under surface with numerous little elevated pale coloured circular dots with a dark centre (indicatiang the points from where the roots arose). The common adulterant of Acorus calamus is orris roots (Iris species) which are readily distinguished by their darker colour different structure and aromatic odour and taste. Phizomes are collected during autumn and early spring.

Current Market Rate : Rhizomes Rs. 20-22 per kg.

Used : Powdered roots are used as vermifnge, Rhizomes are emetic is large doeses, stomachic and carminative is smaller doses; useful is bronchitis and remithent fever. It is a simple and useful remedy for flatuleuce colic or dyspepia and a pleasant adjunct to tonic or purgative medicines. The rootstock and leaves are used in preparation of perfumes and hair powders and for flavouring liquors, beer, vinegar snuff etc. The leaves and roots are also used as an efficacions inseticide for the control of household pests and of insects attacking field crops, stored grains, and wollens. The fresh rootstock is used in confectionery and as a substitute for ginger. Fresh rhizome is inhaled allergic and small pieces if chewed empty stomach help in curing asthma (Manandhar, 1980, chauhan, 1984).

Preparations

(i) Bucha-churna,

(ii) Sarasvata-churna,

(iii) Ashwagandha-rishta,

(iv) Yagaraja-ganggulu,

(v) Sanjivani-vati,

(vi) Chandraprabhavati,

(vii) Unmadgajakesari,

(viii) Mahashankhavati.

Cultivation notes : Clayey leoms and light alluvial soils are suitable for its cultivation. Thefield is irrigated and ploughed with green manure before planting. The growing ends or tops of the previous years crop are planted at 30 cm apart, leaving the leafy portion well above the ground. The crop is ready for harvesting is about a year. The plants are dugout and tops of the stocke are kept for next plantation. the rhizomes are dried is sun hefore they are marked. An acre of crop yields about 15 quintals of dry marketable rhizomes. (Anonymous, 1948). In subsequent years the crop regenerates itself as some pieces of rhizome which remain is the soil sprout up in the growing sealon.

ADIANTUM VENUSTU M G. DON[17]

Family: ADINATACEAE

Local Common Name(s): (i) Hansraj

Description : A dark horwn fern with times pinnate. Rachis slender, polished, naked, segments rigid, prominently vened and toothed, upper edge rounded, lower cuneate into the petiole. Sori 1-3, large, roundish, placed is a distinct hollow on the upper edge.

Parts used : The whole Plant.

Current Market rate : Rs. 15-25 per kg.

Chemical contents: Contains tannis and mucilage.

Properties and used : It possesses astringent and aromatic properties, is emetic is large doses. tonic, febrifuge and expectorant. In Yunani medicines it is used is ohhthalmia, hydrophobia, tumours, colds, headache and is also considered approdisiac. In chamba (HP), it is pounded and applied to bruises, boils and vitlago the plant is useful as a mild tonic especially during convalescence from fevers. It is also used for the prevention of hair from falling. In Yunani system of medicines, theoil obtained from the plant is applied to piles and tubercular glands and wounds and also to bring out a thorn which has penetrated into the body. A few other species growing is the area are also used is similar manner e.g. A capillus-venerisl, A pedatun L and A Lunulatum.

Preparations: The herb is employed as an ingredient in several AYURVEDIC and UNANI systems of medicines especially is deunatological pharmaceutical preparations.

Cultivation Notes: The plant grows naturally in shady and moist slopes, especially along walls, rock builders with sufficient soil deposition on it, along water channels nalahs, natural springs and village bawlies (Source of drinking water). Similar conditions are required for its plantation under domestication can also be grown as indoor poor plant.

AEGLE MARMELOS (L) CORR.[18]

Family : RUTACEAE

Local Common Name(s) : (i) Bel.

Description : A mediumsiaed, deciduous tree, having strong axillary throns, leaves trifoliate, stalked, alternate; leaflets oblanceolate, crenate, gland dotted; middle leaf is stalked and large while the latter one's sessile. Flovers greenish, fragrant. Fruit is globose with woody shells.

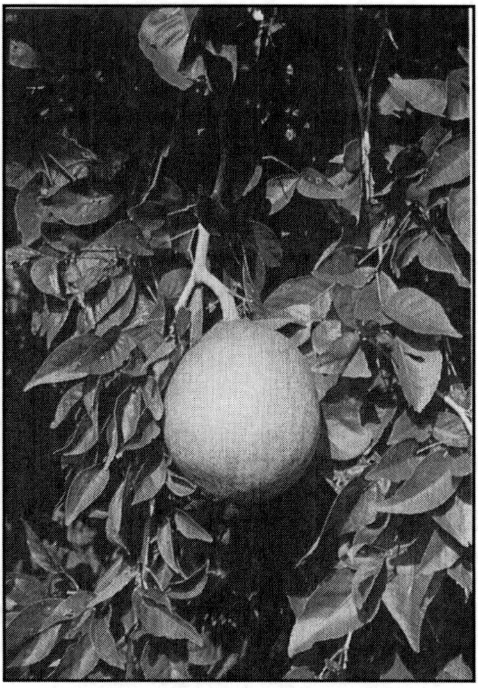

Fig. 2. Bel Aegle Marmelos.

Flowering/Fruiting : Flowers: May - June.

Fruits : May - June of the following year.

Parts used : The ripe and unripe fruits. Fruits are globose and the pulp is mucilaginous aromatic, sweet and astringent. Dried slkes are having on the over side a smooth, greenish-browen shell enclosing a hard orange brown gummy pulp is which cells and seeds may be seen. Dried pulp has a macilaginous, acidic and slightly astringent taste and have agreeable aroma.

Uses : The Bel fruit is valuable chiefly for its macilage and pectin. It is very useful in chronic dysentery diarrhoea, particularly for patients having diarrhoea alternating with spells of consptipation. Sweet drinks (Sharbats) prepared from the pulp of teh fruits are useful as soothing agents for intestines of patients who have just recovered from bacillary dysentery the unripe or half ripe fruits improve appetile and digestion. The antibiotic activity of the leaf fruit and root of this plant has been canfirmed is some recent experiments.

Preparations

(i) Dasmula taila,

(ii) Dasmularista,

(iii) Bilvachuran,

(iv) Gangadhara-Churna,

(v) Amritarista,

(vi) Chyavangprasa,

(vii) Mahanarayana - taila,

(viii) Dhanya panchaka kvatha,

(ix) Pusyanuga churna,

(x) Vatsakadikvatha.

Cultivation Notes: Propagation is through seed which should be taken from ripe fruit on the tree. The seed does not keep well and those in fallen fruits are apt to be useless for sowing. The growth is slow and trees don't start to fruit till they are 5-8 year's is old and are not in full bearing till these are 25-30 year's old. The tree produces root suckers rather freely and these can be used instead of seedlings. Root suckers taken from a good tree are much preferred to seed from an unknown source, if large fruited plants are required.

AESCULUS INDICA COLEBR[19]

Family : HIPPOCASTANACEAF

Local/Common Name(s): (i) Bankhor

Parts used : Seeds.

Current Market Rate: Not Available.

Main Ingredients : The seeds contain a mixture of saponins, one of which is described as aescine, which easily crystailises. Also contains flavonoid glycosides, aesculine, alhumin and fatty oils. (Anonymous, 1948).

Uses: Aesculine is used medically and extracts from the seeds are used industrially. As medicine it is especially used for the complaints of the veins, such as phlelcitis, haemorrhoids, Varicose veins, ulcers; to prevent thromliosis, in some cases of migrains, effusions of blood; for limb complaints and frost bite. Fruits are given to horses in colic, oic from the seeds is extermally applied is rheumatism. the hydroxycoumaringlycoside aesculin from the hark of the branch absorbs ultra-violet rays and is an ingredient for suntan oil (chopraetal, 1956; inanandhar, 1980)

Preparations: Suntan oil and veterinary formulations. Presently, the seeds are being used in the preparation of shampoo.

Cultivation Notes: Can be easily raised through seeds sown is nursery and transplanted. Seeds are collected during October - December and dried in shade after removing the fruit coat. The seeds should not bestored as they are attacked by moulds and insects and should be immediately sown is well prepared nurseries at a distance of 20x10 cm (30 cm apart with seed spaced at 25 cm apart). The seed can best be sown in drills insunkenbeds during October - November before snowfall. 80 - 90 per cent qermination in reported and the seedlings are roady for transplantation after 1 Year.[3]

Weedings are required in the nursery. (Ghosh, 1977, sharma and Sharma, 1988).

AJUGA BRACTEOSA WALL, EX BERTH[20]

Family: LAMIACEAE (LABIATAE)

Local/Common Name(s): (i) Neelkanthi

Description: A perennial, erect or ascending hairy herb, often prostrate, with oblanceolate or subspathulate, obture sinuate toothed leaves; purplish violet tinged from lower surface. Flowers are purplish - violet, tinged from lower surface in distant, axillary whorls in a spike.

Flowering/fruiting: April - October

Parts used: The herbcchiefly leaves

Current Market Rate : Rs. 15 - 25 per kg.

Uses : The aromatic leaves are regarded as stimulat, diuretic, tonic and apparient. It is sand to be a bitter as tringent given in the treatment of fevers and also used as fell rifuge. As an aromatic tonic, it is useful in ague. Also used to kill Lice, regarded as depurative and useful is cases of material fever as a substitute for cinchona; welth of India 1:42; karnick and gout, rheumatism, palsy and amenorr hoea. Ethyl aecobal extract has been found to have anticavcer activity.

Preparations: Mostly consumed in traditional medicines locally and also in AYURVEDIC formulations.

Cultivation : Thouguit occurs as a seasonal weed frequently, yet, if required can be propagated through seeds and by transplanting naturally raising seedlings in appropriate spacings and adopting required cultural operations like application of fertilise rs irrigation, hoeing and weeding.

ALBIAIA LEBBEK BENTH[21]

Family : LEGUMINOSEAE (MIMOSACEAE).

Local/Common Name(s) : (i) Shirish.

Description : The tree is common throughout India, much planted as avenue tree and also in tea gardens for shade (Dey, 1980). It occurs scattered is mixed deciduous forests and ascends to 1200 m is the Himalaya. (Chowdhery and wadhwa, 1984). In Himachal Pradesh, it is found growing is Nauni (1200 m). Nalagarh-Ramshahar, (up to 1200 m) Nahan Division, Kangrg Chambal, Una, Hamirpur, Bilaspur, Maudi, beeov 1,100 m. Also found planted at many places (Chauhan N.S, 1571, 1574, 1884).

Flowering/Fruiting: April-May; pods ripon during September-Octover and remain on the tree for a considerable time.

Parts used : Bark, Leaves, Flower and Seeds.

Current market rate: Not available.

Uses: Siris is considered as alternatives aphrodisiac, astringent, expectorant, restorative and tonic.It is effective is asthma reduces enlargement of cervical gland; is cough and cold; strengthens gums, Thickens and retains seminal fluid. The seed are used in the treatment of piles and as an astringlmt in diarrhoea. The flowers are employed to cure boils, eruptions, swellings and act as antidote to poisons. Leaves are useful in ophthalmia. the powdered hark is useful in ulcers and in snake - bite wounds. Oil obtained from the seeds is useful in leucoderma power of shoot hark strenghens gums. The wood is durable of light colour and fairly strong. It is excellent for high class furnituers interiov decoration and is also much used for house building agriculture implements, rollers, the oil and sugar cane mills, wellcurbs boats, carts, carriages and toys manufacturing. (A nonymous, 1948) the bark is used for tannin and dyeing and as detergent.

Preparations

(i) Mahasirisagad,

(ii) Sirisarishta,

(iii) Dashanglepa.

Cultivation Notes: It can be grownly line sowing on well losened soil, 15-20 cm apart. The tree prefers moistsituations and is found to grow is a variety of soil conditions. Seeds can be collected during January-Inarch and sown during Feb-March. Seeds have to be immersed in hoiling water for 24 hours before sowing in the nursery or polythone bags. Germination is observed to be 60-90 per cent. Trams planting is done during rainy season. Trans plantation of nursery plants and propgation by cuttings are both satisfactory. The rate of growths is very rafid (Anonymous, 1948; Sharma and Sharma, 1988).

ALLIUMSATIVUM LINN[22]

Family: ALLACEAE

Local/Common Name(s) : (i) Lahsun

Description : An annual or perennial, bulbous plant with numerous white bulbs called as cloves enclosed is a commons, membranous white or pinkish covering/sheath. It has long, flat narrow leaves and bears small white flowers and bulbils in a globose mass on a solid scape.

Flowering/Fruiting: May-July.

Parts used: Bulbs.

Current Market Rate: Rs. 40 - 45 per kg.

Properties and uses: As a medicine, garlic was held is high esteam by the ancient physicians of India. it is considered hot and stimulant and is administered in fevors, Coughs and other debiliatating conditions. It has also a reputation as febrifuge in intermitent fevers. Externally, the juice is used as rubefacient in skin diseases and as ear drops in earache and deafness. It is also used in fairly large quantities in western medicines. Various proprietary preparations of garlic have been given in pulmonary phthisis, bronchiactasis, gangvene of the lung and whooping cough. Laryngeal tuberculosis and dyodenal ulcers are treated by garlic juice. Inhalation of the fresh Juice is useful in Pulmonary tuberculosis. It has been found useful in a tonic dyspepsia, flatulence and colic. The Juice diluted with water can be used as a lotion for washing wounds and foululcers. Recently, the garlic pills (pearls) are extensively and effectively used is high blood pressure. It has been found to lower the blood cholesterol. Garlic juice is larvicidal agtainst coulex mosquito. The oil of garlic is appreciated as flavouring agent for meat preparations, soups, canned goods and table sauces (Martingale; 600; watt, 173; chopra et al, 1958; 273-74; Guenther, 6:69). Garlic has proved to be an antibiotic antiseptic, anti diabetic, antiarthritic, anticholesteremic, anti canleer, antibacterial antifungal, insecticidal and pesticidal.

Preparations

(i) Rason - Vati,

(ii) Rason - pind,

(iii) Rasonashtka,

(iv) Lapsundyaghrita,

(v) Garlic capsules and Garlic pearls.

Cultivation : Frequently cultivated for its use as condiment an spice all over the country. cloves from the bulbe are planted is well manured fields during September - October and the crop is harvested during April- July.

ALOE BARBAD ENSIS MILL[23]

Family: LILIACEAE

Local/Common Name(s) : (i) Kumari

Description : A perennial fleshy plant. Leaves sessible, crowded, lanceolate, erect spreading, spiny toothed at the margin fleshy. Flowers: on a scape, scaly branched and longer than leaves, yellow in colour. Fruit capsule.

Parts used: Fleshyleaves.

Current Market Rate : Rs. 0.70 - 1 - 00 per kg.

Flowering/Fruiting: July - September/October - November.

Uses: The plant is bitter colling, purgative, abortifacient, cathartic, stomachic, hlood purifier, emmenagogne, acternative aphrodisiac, anthelnintic, useful in diseases, and uterine complaints. Fresh juice of leaves used as colling. and fevers. Dried juice is useful in constipation. Pulp is edible as confection vegetable and pickle.

Preparations

(i) Kumaryasava,

(ii) Bhringaamaladitaila

(iii) Kumaryadi-vati,

(iv) Rajapravartain-vati,

(v) Loha-rasayana,

(vi) Aloes compound.

Cultivation notes: A healthy mother plant may have as many as 4-10 suckers. These seedlings are removed from mother plants when they are two months old. They are planted along slopes or on a level ground. The spacing between two plants is 60 cm - 60 cm. weeding is called for once in two months. Watering is necessary for a few days after planting. A good drainagl is necessary as thewaterlogging can lead to the decay of theplants.

The yield can be taken in about are to one and a half years. Roughly, one plant of one and half years old weighs around 5-8 kgs.

Even without moisture, the growth of the plant is not that poor. the plant grows lusuriantly in xeric conditions as well.

ANGELICA GLAUCA EDGEW[24]

Family : UMBELLIFERAE (APIACEAE)

Local/Common Name(s) : (i) Chora.

Description : A, tall, robust, erect, aromatic, peremnial herb 1 to 1.5 m tall with thick, stout, pereunial roots to ck. Roots are brownish, Long, fleshy bronching, thick, annulate, fusiform resinous and pungently aromatic. leaves are pinnatic. divided, the basal ones are ternate pinnate. leaflets oval to irreqularly mucronate, serrate; upper surface dark green, lower glaucous. Flowers white or purple is long stalked compound umbels. Fruit: Glabrous, flattened, oblong 12 × 7 mm. The roots and root stock become thick stock became thick and increase with age.

Flowering/fruiting: July - September.

Parts used: Dried roots and roots to cks.

Current Market rate: Not available.

Uses : The root is pungent aromatic, stomachic, tonic, stimulant, carminative, diphoretic and divretic. It Increases appetite and combined. With tonics, it is given in typhod conditions, bronchitis, flatulence, colic and pain is the stomach. Roots are used as spice and condiment. Alos used in obstinale constipation and biliousness. The aromatic root is a flavouring agent for food etc. Roots are also used is the preparation of gin and the liqueurs knawn as bitters (Khory and Katrak, 1948, Mchra et al 1969. Mahauwari and singh, 1965; chopra et al, 1974; chauhan, 1948).7

Preparations: Beside indigenous preparations, it is used in dry gin blending.

Cultivation notes : Can easily be cultivated through seeds. It prefers deep soil, rich is organic matter and partial shade. It can also be raised by making splits/divisions of the collar with vegetative buds along with root.

ARCTIUM LAPPALINN[25]

Family : ASTERACEAE/COMPOSITAE.

Local/Common Name(s)

(i) Jangli kuth

Description: An erect branched, biemnial to perennial. up to 1 m or more tall. Leaves ovate, cordate, margins undulate, usually cottony beneath stalked, 75-30 cm across. Flower heads globose, 1.8 - 3.7 cm across, is terminal clusters. In volucral bracts with riaid aur-like spreading harbed tips. corolla and stamens purple-pink. style white, Achenes oblong ribbed, angled.

Flowering/Fruiting : June-September.

Parts used : Root.

Current Market Rate: Not Available.

Chemical Contents: Main Coustituents are acetic acid, butyric acid, caffeic acid, chlorogenic acid, palmitic acid, propionic acid, stearic acid and tiglic acid; aldepydes, (Acetaldehyde, benzaldehyde, by tyraldehyde, isovaleraldehyde, propionaldehyde and valeraldehyde); Carbohydrates insulin (up to 45-50%), mucilage and pectin suggrs. Other constituents are fats (0.4-0.8%) fixed and voltile oils (0.07 - 0.18%) bitters (lappatin), resintannins etc. Leaves yield germacranolids, bitter sesquiterpenes, lactone, arctiopicrin, fulcinone, arcitol and taraxasterol. Seeds yeld sesquilignans and fruit yield arctin arctigenin, mateiresinol and lappaol.

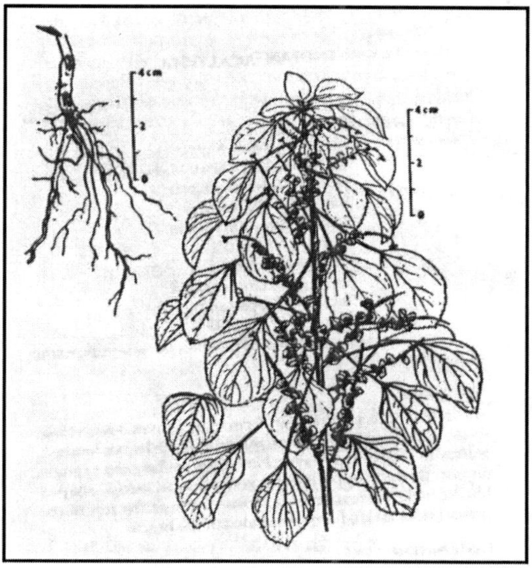

Fig. 3. Indian Acalypha (Acalypha Indica).

Properties and uses : It has diuretic and arexigenic properties and it has been used for cutaneous eruptions, rheumatism, cytitis, gout and specifically for eczema and psoriasis. The plant expact has been found to cause sharp, long lasting requcpion of blood sugar with increuse in carbohydrate tolerance and less toxicity. 50 per cent ethyl alcopol extract was found as cardiac stimulant, diuretic and spasmolytic.

Preparations: It is an official drug of British pharmacopoea used is tumor growth in hillitory mixtures, Liquid Compositions for treating psoriasis and seborrthoic eczemas.

Cultivations notes: It can easily be cultivated through seeds, which have very high germination capacity. Other requirements are same as for SAUSSUREA COSTUS with the added advantage that the former is not successful is monsoon proneareas, where as the later farnishes well in temperate regions with good rainfall.

ARNEBIA BENTH AMI (WALL, EX. G. DON) JOHNSTON SYN. MACROTOMIA BENTHAMI D.C.[26]

Family : BORAGINACEAE.

Local/Common Name(s) : (i) Ratanjot.

Description : An erect. robust herhaceous pereunial, 30-90 cm tall with stout, woody, deep-red roots. Leaves narrow, Lanceolate, hairy. Radical Leaves are large, 28 cm × 1.3 cm; cauline leaves, 7.5 cm.

Flowers pink purple in dense terminal spikes, handing downwards like a tail.

Flawering / Fruiting : July - August.

Parts used : The roots.

Current market rate : Rs. 55.50 per kg.

INDIAN ACALYPHA[27]

Acalypha Indica L.

Family : Euphorbiaceae

Indian names : Hindi-*Khokali, Kuppi.*

Description : An annual herb, up to about 75 cm high. Leaves 3-8 cm long, ovate, thin, usually 3-nerved; margins of the leaves toothed; leafstalks longer than leaves. Flowers in axillary erect spikes; female flower supported by conspicuous wedge-shaped bracts, male flowers; male flowers, minute, brone towards the top of the spike. Fruits small, hairy, concealed in the bracts.

Distribution : The plant is found almost throughout India in the plains; it grows as a weed in gardens and agricultural fields or as a plant iof waste places and on road sides.

Drug and its Properties : The whole plant of this herb collected in its flowering stage; and dried, constitutes the drug *Acalypha.*

The properties of this drug resemble those of *Ipecae.* It is useful in bronchitis, asthma, pneumonia and rheumatism. Its roots and leaves have laxative properties. Juice of leaves is considered an efficient emetic, that is, a medicine for causing vomiting. A poultice of fresh leaves is useful on ulcers.

ACONITE[28]

Aconitum Species

Family : Ranunculaceae

Indian names : *Aconitum chasmanthum* Stapf ex Holmes : Kashmiri-*Mohri*

The drug *Aconite* comprises tuberous roots of these plants; it has been well-known in medicine as it possesses certain very toxic and poiisonous substances. The British Pharmacopoeia recognises the drug obtained from A. *napellus* L. This species in not found in India; but Indian species contain similar substances or are suitable substitues.

A.*heterophyllum (Atis)* is a herb occurring in higher ranges of north-western Himalayas at altitudes of about 2,000 to 4,000 m. The drug obtained from this species is least toxic, it is used in fevers and post-fevers. weakness, diarrhoea and dysentery. Its utility as a tonic has now been recognised but it is not regarded very useful in fevers.

A. *chasmanthus (Banbalnag)* occurs in name regions as *Aist.* The *Aconite* obtained from this plant is considered a suitable substitute for the *Aconite* obtained from A. *napellus.* Though the total alkaloid content of *Banbalnag* is about ten times that of the European Aconite, the potency of the drug is not as good.

A. *deinorrhizum* and a few species of *Aconitum* occur in India and are considered to be of restricted medicinal use.

The alkaloids contained in *Aconites* are very toxic, and unless given in properly controlled doses, can cause dangerous side-effects.

Plants form mountainous regions are more rich in aconitine; the toxicity is due to compounds other than acnitine. Due to the toxic effects, the drug is administered in properly controlled doses. The chief usage of the drug now is only for external application in diseases like neuralgia.

CALAMUS[29]

(Sweet-flag)

Acorus Calamus L.

Family : Araceae.

Indian names : Hindi-*Bach, Ghorabach, Safed-bach.*

Description : A herbaceoun plant with long, creeping and much-branched aromatic rhizomes. Flowering shoots supported by a large leaflike structure spathe. Flowers small, pale-green, in 5-10 cm long cylindric spikes called spadix; fruits yellowish in colour.

Distribution : bracts, present on the spikes; these are conspicuously veined. Corolla (the whorl of petals) of the flowers is white with few purplish markings. Fruits capsular, 4-seeded.

Distribution : This plant occurs throughout the plains and submontane regions of India; it is common near habitations.

Drug and its Properties : The drug *Vasaka* comprises the fresh or dried leaves of the plant. Leaves contain an alkaloid vasicine, and an essential oil. The chief use of *Vasaka* is as an expectorant; it is given in the from of juice, syrup or decoction. It softens the thick sputum, facilitates its coming out and thus brings about quick relief in bronchitis. The expectorant activity is due to stimulation of bronchial glands. Larger doses can, however, cause irritation and vomiting. Recent experiments have confirmed the usefulness of *Vasaka*.

Other Uses : The leaves of this plant are also utilised as green manure and for yielding a yellow dye. Due to the presence of certain alkaloids, the leaves are not easily attacked by fungi and insects, and are, therefore, used in packing or storing fruits. The leaves emit an unpleasant smell and are spared from browsing; the plant is, therefore, suitable for planting in soil reclamation programmes.

GREATER GALANGAL[30]

(Java Galangal, Galangal Major)

Alpinia Galanga (L.) Willd.

Family : Zingiberaceae.

Indian names : Hindi-*Kulinjan, Sugandhbach.*

Description : A herbaceous plant up 2 m high; leaves long, narrow, green above, pale beneath, whitish on margins, median nerve very strong. Flowers about 3 cm long, greenish white; in compound dense bunches; lip of corolla white, streaked with red. Fruit orange-red, size of a small cherry. Rhizomes slightly aromatic.

Distribution : The plant occurs naturally in the eastern Himalayas and the Western Ghats; it is also cultivated at several places.

Drug and its Properties : *Greater Galangal* is the dried rhizome of this plant.

It is useful in rheumatism, respiratory complaints specially of children, and in bronchial catarrh. The drug is also considered useful in stomach complaints and as a tonic, deodorant and disinfectant. It is a stimulant aromatic like ginger.

Other Species : Another important species of the genus *Alpinia* is *a. officinarum* hance *(Lesser Galangal);* it is a native of China. The rhizomes obtained from the chinese species have stronger odour and taste. The plant is extensively cultivated in bengal and northern India.

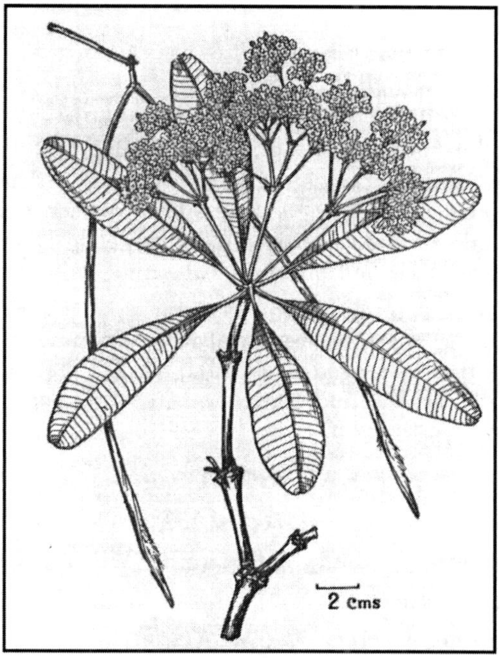

Fig. 4. Chhatim Alstonia Scholaris.

CHHATIM[31]

Alstonia Scholaris (L.) R. Br.

Family *:* Apocynaceae

Indian names : Hindi-*Chhatin.*

English name *:* Devil's tree.

The trade name is based on the more common Indian name for the plant. The Sanskrit name refers to 7 leaves in a whorl.

Description : A large evergreen tree reaching up to about 25 m high: having bitter milky juice; bark rough, dark grey; branches whrled; base of the tree often fluited or buttressed. Leaves lethery, 10-20 cm long, 4-7 in a whorl. Flowers small, greenish white, spice-scented in many-flowered clusters. Fruits very long, 30-60 cm, narrow and slender, hanging in pairs and forming dense clusters.

Distribution : This tree is found in the more moist regions throughout the country.

Drug and its Properties : *Chhatims* is the dried bark of the tree

This drug is considered very efficacious in chronic dlarrhoea and dysentery. It is useful in malarial fever and brings down the temperature gradually and without causing perspiration or exhaustion, which usually follow other medicines for malaria.

***Chhatim* is useful also in skin diseases :** The drug is reported to cause paralysing effect on the motor nerves and consequent fall in blood pressure. Some experiments have contradicted antibiotic and physiological activity of the drug.

Other Uses : The wood of the tree is used for inferior quality furniture, packing cases, tea boxes, pencils and matchsticks. The timber of the tree was used in olden times for making wooden slates *(takhti)* for school children; this was the origin of the specific name *scholaris* for the plant.

KALMEGH[32]

(Andrographis)

Andrographis Paniculata (Burm. f.) Wll. ex Nees

Family : Acanthaceae.

Indian names : Hindi-*Kirayat, Kulufnath.*

(Madhya Pradesh-*Chiretta*).

The trade name *Kalmegh* is taken from the Bengali local name of the plant; and *Andrographis* from the scientific name.

Description : An erect branched annual herb, branches sharply four-angled. Leaves lance-shaped. Flowers small, in large, spreading and sparse bunches. Flowers rose-coloured, about 1cm long. Fruit capsular, 1.5-2 cm.

Distribution : The plant occurs throughout India, chiefly in the plains.

Drug *Kalmegh* Consists of all parts of the plant above ground, i.e. excluding only the roots.

Kalmegh is a bitter tonic, it is useful in curing fever, worms, dysentery, general weakness and excessive gas formation in stomach. It is also reported to be useful for children suffering from liver and digestion complaints.

In Bengal, a household medicine, claled 'Alui' is prepared form its leaves, it is given to babies suffering from stomach complaints.

There had been a belief that this plant was useful also in snake-bite; experiments found this claim to be unfounded. Experiments have shown that the plant has antityphoid and antibiotic properties.

(The tribals of Bastar pound the plant in mustard *(Sarson)* oil and apply on itching).

INDIAN BIRTHWORT[33]

(Aristolochia)

Aristolochia Indica L.

Family : Aristolochiaceae.

Indian names: Hindi-Isharmul, Ishwari.

The trade names are based on the common English name and the scientific name of the plant.

Description : A twining shrub. Stems woody below, slender and soft above. Main rootstock woody. Leaves variable in size and shape form linear, that is, very narrow, to obovate, that is, broader towards tip. Flowers small, greenish-white, in small bunches arising from the axil of the leaves. Flowers purple, characteristically trumpet-shaped. Fruit about 5 cm long, longer than broad, opening from below upwards into six valves.

Distribution : It is found throughout India in lower hilly regions and in plains; it is more common in southern and eastern India.

Drug and its Properties : *Aristolochia* consists of the dried stems and roots of the plant. This drug is useful only in very controlled doses; in small doses it promotes digestion and regulates menstruation; it is a tonic. In largeer doses it causes dangerous irritations in the digestive system and in kidneys and leads to violent vomiting, nausea, even abortion and other disorders.

In regulated doses, *Aristolochia* is used also as stimulant and for curing fevers; it also has some effect on blood pressure.

Other Species : Another species of this genus, *Aristolochia bracteolata* Lamk. ***(Gujarati and Hindi-Kiramar, Sanskrit-Dhumrapatra, Kannada-Kurigida, Tamil-Gariore-gurpa-arku)*** occurs in plains throughout India, particularly in hte regions of black-cotton or 'regur' soils, and is considered useful in worms and on foul ulcers.

WORMSEED[34]

(Artemisia)

Artemisia Maritima L.

Family : Asteraceae

Indian names : Hindi-*Kirmani ajvain, Chhuhri ajmud,* Kirmala.

This drug is also called *Santonina;* this refers to the active principles contained in the plants of the genus *Artemisia.*

Description : A stout, much-branched, perennial, aromatic shrub, about 1 m high. Leaves 2-5 cm long, whitish in colour, divided into numerous fine, linear segments: upper leaves simple, un divided linear. Flowear heads small, in short spikes.

Distribution : The plant occurs in northern India from Kashmir to kumaon at about 2,000 to 3,000 m altitude.

Drug and its Properties : The drug consists of the dried immature leaves and flower heads of the plant. It has been recommended that the drug should be collected in early simmer or late spring, by which time the flower heads have not fully matured.

The medicinal properties of this plant are based chiefly on Santonin, contained in the young leaves and flower heads; the proportionof Santonin is reported to be maximum just before the flowers begin to open; it diminishes soon after.

The chief use of the drug is for expulsion of worms (chiefly thread worms and roundworms) from the stomach. The worms are pushed to large bowels, from where they are removed by a purgative. The drug is also useful in fevers and dropsy, and as a stimulant.

Other Species : Several other species of the genus *Aremisisa* are used in medicine. *Artemisia nilagirica.*

(Cl.) Pamp. (Bengali and Hindi-*Nagdona,* Sanskrit-*Nagdamni,* Tamil-*Machipatri)* occurs in hilly regions of India and is used for worms, asthma, etc. A. *absinthium* L. *(Afsanthin)* occurs in Kasnmir and is useful as a tonic and digestive.

The need for expanding cultivation of Santonin-yielding species of *Artemisia,* in India has been suggested from time to time.

Artemisia species can be grown in the inner ranges of the Himalayas in Kashmir, Punjab, Himachal Pradesh, and Uttar Pradesh, at altitudes of about 2,000 to 3,000 m.

BELLADONNA[35]

Atropa Acuminata Royle ex Lindley

Family : Solanaceae.

Indian names : Hindi-*Angurshafa, Sagangur.*

The trade name *Belladonna (or Indian Belladonna)* is derived from the scientific anme of another species of *Atropa,* namely *A. belladonna* L., which occurs in Europe, and is found in India only under cultivation.

Description : An erect, branched perennial herb, 60-90 cm high. Leaves brownish green, 7-15 cm long, narrowed at both ends. Flowers in axils of leaves, solitary or in paris, about 2.5 cm long, bell-shaped, yellowish brown. Berry roundish, about 1.5 cm across, purple-black.

Distribution : It is found in Kashmir at altitudes of 2,000 to 3,500 m. It is also cultivated.

Drug and its Properties : The drug *Belladonna* Consists of the dried leaves and other aerial parts of the plant; roots are also included.

Total alkaloid content depends upon stage of development of plant, low during flowering and very high when bearing green berries.

The drug obtained from the leaves and other aerial parts brings about a decrease in secretion of sweat and salivary and gastric glandds; it acts as strong anti-spasmodic in intestinal colic and other spasmodic indications. It is also useful in asthma and whooping cough.

The drug obtained from the root of the plant has similar properties as the one obtained from leaves and twigs. Roots, are however, belived ot have certain poisonous substances and are employed chiefly in preparation prescribed for external applications on rheumatism, neuralgia, inflammations, etc.

Other Species : Another important species of this genus, namely *Atropa beladonna* (L.) (Deadly nightshade) is a native of Europe and is cultivated in hilly regions of India. Its roots (called *Belladonna radix* in commerce) and leaves (called *Belladonna folium)* are of medicinal importance, chiefly as tonic, antispasmodic and sedative, the precise use depending on dosage. It has the property of dilating pupils of eyes, and its preparations (like Atropine) have been largely employed as eye-drops or ointments

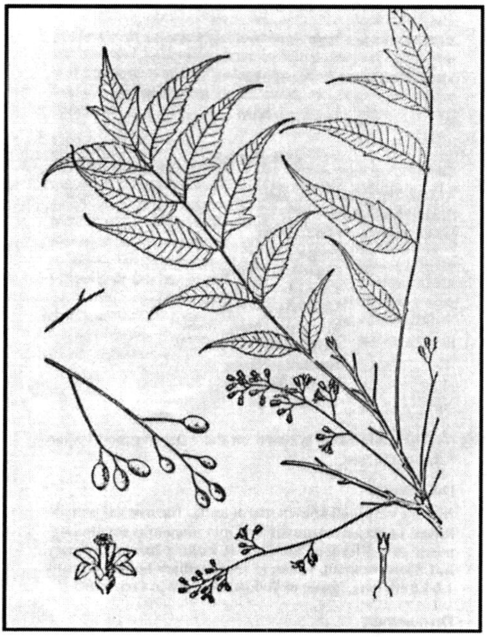

Fig. 5. Nim (Azadirachta Indica).

used at the time of testing the eyes and other ophthalmic treatments. It is useful as an antidote in certain types of poisoning cases.

NIM[36]

(Margosa tree)

Azadirachta Indica A. Juss.

Family : Medliaceae.

Indian names : Hindi-*Nim.*

The trade name is based on the most common Indian name of the tree.

Description : *Nim* is a very well-known tree of India. The tree has pinnate leaves, i.e. its leaves are divided into numerous smaller segments called leaflets, each leaflet looking like an ordinary leaf. Flowers small, white, in short axillary bunches. Fruit.

Distribution : The tree occurs naturally in Deccan Peninsula, but is cultivated all over India near habitations and on road sides, etc.

Drug and its Properties : The drug consists of dried stem bark, leaves, and bark.

The bark is a bitter tonic, astrringent and antiperiodic, i.e. it is useful in fevers, it breaks the periodic sequence of fevers (like malaria) and is useful in skin diseases.

The antibiotic activity of leaves and roots of the tree and their utility in skin diseases have been confirmed experimentally.

Other Uses : The timber of *Nim* tree is very durable and is useful for house building, agricultural implements and miscellaneous carpentry work. The oil cake and gum which exudate from bark are also useful products. Dried leaves are placed among clothes to keep moths away.

BRAHMI[37]

(Bacopa)

Bacopa Monnieri (L.) Penn syn. *Herpestis monniera* (L.) H.B.K., *Monnicra cuneifolia* Mich.

Family : Scrophulariaceae

Indian names : Hindi-*Brahmi. Safed Chamni.*

English name : Thyme-leaved Gratiola.

The trade names *Brahmi* and *Bacopa* are based on the local Indian and scientific names of the plant respectively.

Description : This herb spreads on ground and its stems and small leaves are succulent, i.e. fleshy. Roots arise on the nodes of the stem also. Flowers arise in the axils of the leaves and are borne on short pedicels. One of the five sepals is larger than others. The corolla is bluish-white in colour and about 1 cm across.

Drug and its Properties : The drug *Barhmi* consists of the whole plant.

It is valued in medicine as a tonic for nerves and is prescribed in nervous disorders (accompanied by convulsions or unconsciousness), mental diseases, constipation and as a diuretic, i.e. to promote urination. Leaf juice is given to infants in bronchitis; the relife is due to the vomiting and purging brought about by the drug. Leaf juice, mised with petroleum, is applied on rheumatism. A poultice made of the boiled plant is placed on the chest of children suffering from cough. The plant is consdered a blood purifier.

The tranquillising efect of the alcholic extract of this plant has been successfully tested on animals experimentally. The plant contains an alkaloid Bramhine, which is a cardiac tonic, i.e. provides strength and tone to the heart.

INDIAN BARBERRY[38]

(Berberis)

Berberis Aristata DC.

Family *:* Berberidaceae.

Indian names : Hindi : *Daru-haldi, Kngora, Kilmora, Rasaut.*

Description : A large throny shrub; wood yellow; branches whitish or pale grey. Leaves characteristic, fascicled in axils of branched or simple spines, coriaceous, usually sharp-toothed, veins very fine. Flowers yellow, in short bunches. Fruit ovoid, bluish purple; seeds few.

Drug and its Properties *: Berberis* consists of dried roots of this plant and also of certain other closely related plants belonging to the same genus, e.g. *B. asiatica* Roxb. and *B. lycium* Royle.

The chief constituent of the drug is the alkaloid Berberine.

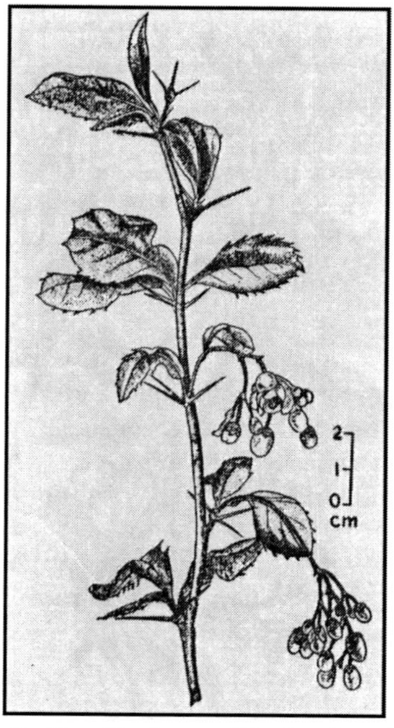

Fig. 6. Indian Barberry (Berberis aristata)

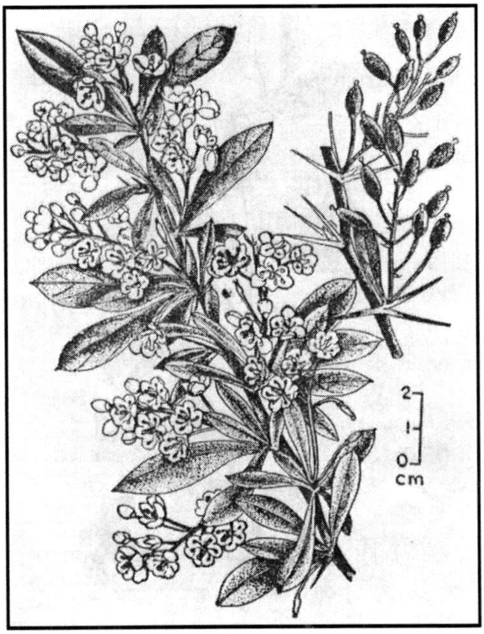

Fig. 7. Indian Barberry (Berberis lycium).

Root bark, roots and lower stems are boiled in water, strained and evaporated till a semi-solid mass is obtained; this is called *Rasaut,* it is fairly soluble in water.

Mixed with butter and alum, or with opium and lime juice, *Rasaut* is applied externally on eye lids to cure ophthalmia and other eye diseases. The use of *Rasaut* in curing ulcers has been shown exerimentally. It is also administered through injections near the margins of the sores.

Rasaut is used in curing fevers, and as mild laxative nad tonic. It is useful in stomach disorders and its experimental use in cholera and acute diarrhoea in rabbits has been confirmed.

The drug was also, for some time, used in malarial fever, but its curative effect has been disproved; it does, however, help in early detection of malarial fever.

The depressant action of the drug on respiration and heart has also been shown experimentally. Antitubercular activity has also ben attributed to this drug.

Other Uses : The root and stem of B. *aristata* yield a yellow dye, which is used for tanning and colouring leather.

PUNARNAVA[39]

Boerhavia Diffusa L.

Family : Nyctaginaceae.

Indian names : Hindi-*Bishkopra, Punarnava, Sant, Santhi, Survari.*

English names : Horse-purslane, Hogweed.

The trade name is based on the Sanskrit name of the plant. In old Indian literature it is referred to as 'Sothaghna' i.e. destroyer of dropsy.

Description : Amuch - branched herb, generally spreading on the ground or partly ascending. Leaves two on each node, one smaller than the other, base of the leaves cordate; lower surface of leaves whitish, upper green. Flowers very small, eddish, in short clusters on long axillary stalks. Fruit with five ridges, glandular.

Distribution : The plant is found in all parts of India.

Drug and its Properties : The whole plant, particularly the roots, leaves and seeds constiute the drug *Punarnava.*

The drug contains the alkaloid, Punarnavine. The main use of the drug is as a diuretic, i.e. to promote urination in dropsy and in jaundice and gonorrhoea. It is also a laxative. In moderate doses, it is recommended for asthma. Large doses can bring about vomiting.

The diuretic activity of the drug has been experimentally confirmed on animals.

BUTEA[40]

(Palas, Flame of the Forest)

Butea Monosperma (Lamk.) Taub. syn. *B. frondosa* Koen. ex Roxb.

Family : Fabaceae.

Indian names : Hindi - *Dhak, Palas, Tesu.*

(Ajmer-Merwara-_Chaura)._

The trade name Butea is based on the scientific name of the plant; *Palas* and *Flame of the Forest* are based on local Indian and English names of the tree respectively.

Description *: Palas* is a well-Known tree of India. Its scarlet and orange flowers come in such profusion that the tree has been very aptly named the *Flame of the Forest.* It is a medium-sized tree with compound leaves, each leaf comprising three leaflets; leaflets silky tomentous and strongly veined on lower surface; the leaves fall off in winter. Flowers appear in about February to March in small but dense clusters generally on leafless branches, and the tree appears to be loaded with a mass of orange colour. The fruit is a flat pod having a single seed. The name *monosperma* refers to the single seed.

Distribution : The tree is found all over India, chiefly in the mixed or dry deciduous forests of central and western India. It is more common in the plains or lower regions of hills.

Drug and its Properties : The red coloured gum, called *Bengal Kino* or *Butea Gum* are obtained from this tree and the seeds of the tree are medicinal.

The gum contains tannins and is valuable for treatment of diarrhoea.

The seeds are used as anthelmintic in treatment of roundworms and tapeworms. Their usefulness in treatment of roundworms has been confirmed through some recent experiments. Seeds of *Butea* are a suitable substitute for *Santonina.* The seeds, pounded with lemon juice, are applied on Dhobi's itch. Seeds are also useful on ringworm. The root bark has been found to have some action on blood pressure.

Other Uses : This tree is highly valued as a host tree for the lacinsect. The flowers yield a yellow dye. The wood lasts well under water and is used for well curbs and water scoops. It is also used for miscellaneous construction work and as fuel. Leaves are largely used for making bowls *(dauna)* and plates *(pattals)* for serving food, and as fodder.

Other Species *: Butea superba* Roxb. (Hindi-*Palas lata)* is a robust woody climber occurring almost throughout India. Its leaf juice is useful in heat eruptions in children.

CASSIA[41]

(Indian Laburnum)

Cassia Fistula L.

Family : Caesalpiniaceae

Indian names : Hindi-*Amaltas, Kilvali, Kirala, Sinar.*

The trade name is based on the scientific name; the specific anme *fistula;* which menas a shepherd's pipe, refers to the shape of the fruit of the tree.

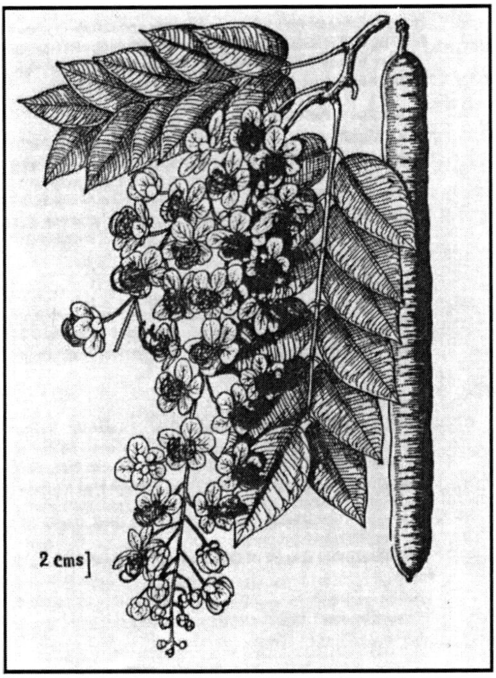

Fig. 8. Cassia (Cassia Fistula).

Description : It is a small or medium-size tree with compound leaves and large, shining, dark green leaflets. Flowers bright yellow, in very large, hanging bunches. Fruits 50-60 cm long, black or shining dark brown, almost cylindric. The tree is a conspicuous sight in flowers as well as in fruits and can be spotted in a forest even from long distance. The tree sheds its leaves during early summer (March-May), and is in full blomm during this period.

Distribution : This tree is found throughout India up to an altitude of about 1,500 m, and is more common in moist or evergreen forests.

The tree is much favoured for planting in road-side avenues and in gardens.

Drug and its Properties : Though medicinal properties have been attributed to nearly all parts of the tree, the fruits are most important and are included in the Indian Pharmaceutical Codex. The pulp from the fruits, called *Cassia pulp,* is a well-known laxative. In larger quantities, it causes purging, nausea and griping.

It is not used singly, but in admixture with *Senna (C.angustifolia)* leaves etc.

Other Uses : The bark of this tree is known as 'Sumari' and is rich in tannins. The timber of the tree is strong and tough and is suitable for house and bridge posts and agricultural implements.

Other Species : *Cassia angustifolia* Vahl (*Indian Senna, Tinneveliy Senna,* Hindi-*Sanai,* Sanskrit-*Bhupadma,* Malayalam-*Nilavaka)* is a small shrub of Arabia and Somaliland and has been successfully cultivated in south India. Leaves and fruits of this plant are cathartic and are useful in habitual costiveness. It is reported that if nursing women take this drug, their milk acquires purgative properties.

Several other species of *Cassia* are of restricted medicinal value.

CATHARANTHUS[42]

(Sadabahar)

Catharanthus roseus (L.) Don syn. *Vinca rosea* L., *Lochnera rosea* (L.) Reichb.

Family : Apocynaceae.

Indian names : Hindi-*Sadabahar.*

(Punjab-*Rattanjot*).

Description : An erect herb up to about 1 m high; leaves ovate, opposite; flowers in axillary clusters of 2 or 3; petals white or rose-pink, in one variety petals white with pink or reddish tinge at base; fruits many-seeded, follicles.

Distribution : The plant is a native of Madagascar, but has become naturalised throughout the tropics of both hemispheres.

Drug and its properties : The roots of the plant constitute the drug. They were known to possess toxic and stomachi properties, but recently they have gained repute as a source of valuable alkaloids resembling those from *Rauvolfia* species. Roots of *Catharanthus* have more ajmalicine and serpentine than even *Rauvolfia serpentina;* they also possess reserpine.

The alkaloids possess hypotensive, sedative and tranquillising properties.

Experiments on anmials have shown that certain extracts of *Chatharanthus* are useful in leukaemia.

Other Uses : The plant is a handsome garden plant and flowers throughout the year; this gives the plant the name 'Sadabahar'. The plant is quite hardy and is popular for ornamental planting.

Other Species : *Catharanthus pusillus* G. Don [Syn. *Vinca pusilla* Murr., *Lochnera Pusilla* (Murr.) K. Schum, Sanskrit-*Sangkhaphuli*, Kannada-*Viskanigalu*, Tamil-*Milagai Poondu*] occurs as a weed, and is reported to be useful in lumbago.

CENTELLA[43]

(Indian Pennywort)

Centella Asiatica (L.) Urban syn. *Hydrocotyle asiatica* L.

Family : Apiaceae.

Indian names: Hindi-*Brahmmanduki, Brihmi, Budhbrahmani.*

The Sanskrit name *Mandukparni* refers to the leaves of the plant which resemble the claw of a frog.

Description : The plant trails on the ground and its creeping stems bear roots on their nodes. Leaves small, 2-4 cm diameter, sometimes more rounded or broak kidney-shaped, their margins toothed. Flowers minute, Pinkish red, 3-6 in cluster. Fruits small, like a grain of barley, 7-9 ridged.

Distribution : This plant grows in moist places throughout India, it is commonly seen in marshy banks of rivers, streams and ponds and in irrigated lawns, fields, etc.

Drug and its Properties : The drug comprises fresh and dried leaves nad stems of this plant. Roots and seeds are also used in medicine.

The leaves or the entire plant parts are boiled in water and this decoction is given in teratment of leprosy.

The plant contains asiaticoside, which is considered responsible for its use in leprosy. Experiments on animals have confirmed its property of inducing fast growth of skin, hair, and nails.

The plant is also considered useful in certain kinds of tuberculosis and as a tonic for brain.

CENTRATHERUM[44]

(Somraj)

Centratherum Anthelminticum (Willd.) Kuntze syn. *Vernonia anthelmintica* Willd.

Family : Asteraceae.

Indian names : Hindi-*Banjira; Somraj, Somraji.*
(Garhwal-*Kala zira.*)

The trade names *Centratherum* and *Somraj* are based on scientific and Sanskrit names of the plant respectivesly. The word *antheiminticum* in the scientific name suggests the medicinal usage of this plant in treatment of worms.

Description : An erect tall herb; stems and leaves covered with minute hairs. Leaves 6-10 cm long, their amrgins toothed, base tapering into a petiole. Flower heads 1.5-2.5 cm diameter, in small clusters, each head with 30-40, minute purplish flowers. Fruits, which are scientifically, called achenes, 4.5-6 mm long, cylindric, hairy with 10 narrow ridges; the tuft of hairs on top of achenes, reddish.

Distribution : This plant is found throughout India up to an altitude of about 1,500 m, and is more common in waste places near habitations.

Drug and its Properties : The drug comprises fresh (as fresh as possible) dried seeds of the plant.

As the scientific name of the plant indicates, it is a valuable medicine as anthelmintic, that is, to destroy worms. It is useful in thread worm infections.

In old literature, the plant has been reported to be useful also as a stimulant and antiseptic and for promoting urination, but experiments have shown it to be almost ineffective in these respects. Its utility in thread worm infections has been confirmed in trials in hospitals.

IPECAC[45]

(Ipecacuanha)

Cephaelis Ipecacuanha (Brot.) A. Rich.

Family : Rubiaceae.

Description : A small trailing herb. Roots slender, spreading horizontally. Mature roots moniliform, in bunches. Leaves in opposite pairs, their tips pointed, margins entire. Flowers white, small, in small bunches.

Distribution : This plant is a native of Brazil in South America and is cultivated in India in Assam, Bengal and on an experimental scale in South India.

Drug and its Properties : The rhizomes of the plant constitute the drug *Ipecac.*

This drug is useful in amoebic dysentery and loss of appetite; given in larger doses, it brings about vomiting and this property is utilised for bringing relief in cough. It also acts as a diaphoretic, i.e. brings about sweating.

The Ipecac plantation in West Bengal has been developed as the largest in the world, and India's internal requirement is now amply met from this plantation. The Ipecac root has great export potential, and expansion of its cultivation has been recommended.

CINCHONA[46]

Cinchona species.

Family : Rubiaceae.

Indian names : The commonest local name is *Kunain,* it is based on *quinine,* the main active principle in the bark of *Cinchona* trees.

The trade name is based on the scientific name *Cinchona.*

The genus *Cinchona* is not indigenous to India, and none of its species occur here in natural state. Several species are, however, now cultivated in India; four of them are more important. These are :

1. *Cinchona calisaya* Wedd. (Trade name: *Calisaya Bark, peruvian Bark).* it is cultivated in Nilgiris and Sikkim.
2. *C. ledgeriana* Moens (Trade name: *Ledger Bark).* It is grown in Bengal, Assam and South India, and is the commonest *Cinchona* gown in India.
3. *C. officinalis* L. (Trade name : *Crown Bark, Loxa Bark).* It is grown in Nilgiris.
4. *C. succirubra* Pav. ex klotzsch (Trade name; *Red Bark).* It is grown in Satpura hills, Sikkim and South India.

Cinchona species grown in India are usually large or medium-sized trees; *C. ledgeriana* is a straggling tree.

Drug and its Properties : The dried bark of the above mentioned species constitutes the drug *Cinchona.*

Cinchona bark yields several active principles, of which quinine is most important; it is well-known for its effevtive use in malarial fevers. The drug causes quick remission of fever and with repeated or regulated doses, checks relapse of malarial fevers. Quinine also destroys certain infections, and in certain preparations has been found useful in pneumonia, amoebic dysentery and for eye lotions.

Preparations of quinine are also useful as local applications on certain rheumatic pains and as gargles.

Higher doses of quinine preparations can cause temporary (or even permanent) deafness, blindness, giddiness and nausea. Pregnant women and persons with heart ailments are not given quinine preparations.

Other Uses : Preparations based on quinine and on other active principles of *Cinchona* bark have been used as insecticides for preservation of feathers, furs, clothes, etc., as moth repellants, and even as hair lotions.

The *Cinchona* bark from which quinine has been extracted, serves as a tanning material.

CINNAMON[47]

Cinnamomum Verum Presl. Syn. *C. zeylanicum* Blume.

Family : Lauraceae.

Indian names : Hindi-*Dalchini.*

Description : It is an evergreen tree, i.e. it does not become totally leafless at any time of the year; about 6-8 m high. Leaves large, ovate, thick, leathery, pointed at tip, shining green, lighter coloured beneath; main nerves on the leaves 3 ro 5, running from base of leaf to middle or tip. Flowers minute, in large hairy clusters. Fruits oblong or ovate, about 1.5-2 cm long, dark purple, seed one.

Distribution : This tree occurs in South India up to an altitude of about 1,500 m, is more common at lower altitudes, even below 200 m. It is also cultivated in certain other parts of India.

Drug and Its Properties : The branches of the trees are lopped and their bark removed; the dried inner bark constitutes the drug *Cinnamon.*

The drug is used in diarrhoea, nausea, and vomiting. It is commonly used as condiment.

The oil obtained from the bark, called Cinnamon bark oil has similar properties, and even has certain advantages over the bark.

It is used as a stomachic and carminative, it cures gastric debility and flatulence; and also has the property of destroying certain germs and fungi.

Other Uses : The oil obtaind from leaves is used as a flavouring agent and preservative for sweets, soaps, etc., and for local application on certain rheumatic pains. South India, Bengal,

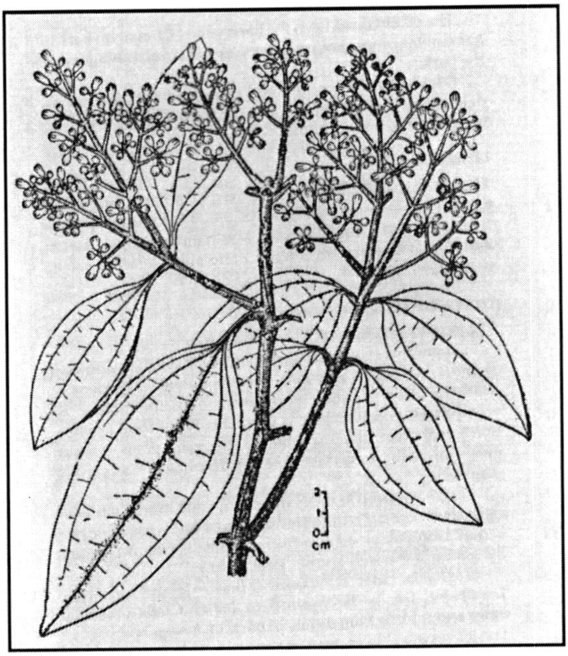

Fig. 9. Cinnamon (Cinnamomum Verum).

Assam and Andamans are considered more suitable areas for its cultivation.

Other Species : The genux *Cinnamomum* has several other useful species.

C. *camphora* (L.) Presl (Camphor tree, *Kapur)* is cultivated in India in Nilgiris and also in some botanical gardens of northen India. *Camphor* is obtained by disillation of its wood and leaves. *Camphor* is used chiefly for local application on sprains, inflammations and rheumatic pains. It is also given internally in certain types of diarrhoea or as cardiac stimulant.

Camphor is used in many other ways and more than 5,000 quintals of *Camphor* is imported into India each year. *(Camphor* is now being obtained also from certain species of *Ocimum,* the genus of the well-known *Tulsi* plant).

C. teamala Nees and Eberm. (Hindi-*Tejpat,* Sanskrit-*Tamalpatra,* Tamil-*Talishpattiri)* or *Indian Cassia* occurs in outer and middle Himalayas, in parts of Assam and Bengal. The leaves are chiefly used as a spice, but also as a carminative and in colic and diarrhoea.

COLCHICUM[48]

Colchicum Luteum Baker.

Family: Liliaceae.

Indian names : Hindi-*Hirantutiya.*

The trade name is dervied from the scientific name. Two articles from this plant, viz. seeds and corms (fleshy underground stems), are articles of commerce and are called *Colchicum seed* and *Colchicum corm* respectively.

Description : An annual herb; corms brownish in colour, almost conical in shape, with one side flat, the other roundish. Leaves very narrow but broade towards the tip, increasing in size as the plant approaches fruiting stage, 15-30 cm long, 0.8-1.5 cm broad, Flowers large, 2.5-4 cm diameter, 7-10 cm long, their beaks recurved.

Distribution : The plant is found in north-western Himalayas from about 700 to 2,800 m altitude, usually in outskirts of forests or in open grassy places.

Drug and its Properties : The fresh corms of the plant collected before its flowering constitute the drug *Colchicum corm,* and the ripe dried seeds, the drug *Colchicum seed.*

The corms contain the active principle Colchicine. It is useful in pains and inflammations of gout. Clinical experiments with *Colchicum* in small doses over a long period have shown sucess in about sixty per cent of patients. The use of the drug can, however, cause sever irritation in intestines and to counteract this, the use of the drug with *Belladonna* or *Hyoscyamus* is recommended.

The seeds, chiefly the seed-coat (rind), also contain Colchicine. The drug is useful in the same manner as the corms.

The effect of Colchicine on cancerous tissues has been tested and it has been shown that the drug arrests division of cells of the cancerous tissues and also makes them more susceptible to X-ray treatments. Experiments on these prospects are still continuing in certain research institutes, and the drug has not yet been put in actual use.

The plant can be grown at higher altitudes (1,500-3,000 m) in the Himalayas.

Other Uses : Colchicine has been largely used in scientific research in plant breeding; it induces polypolidy, that is, multiplication of basic chromosome numbers.

COPTIS[49]

Coptis Teeta Wall.

Family: Ranunculaceae.

Indian names : Hindi-*Mamira, Mishmi tita.*

Description : A small stemless herb; root-stock woody, golden yellow, densely fibrous, very bitter. Leaves compound, glabrous, leaflets 5.0-7.5 cm long, ovate, lanceolate, pinnatifid. Flowers 1-3, small, regular, white; fruit many-seeded follicles; seeds black.

Distribution : Temperate regions of Mishmee hills in Arunachal Pradesh in India.

Drug and its Properties : The dried rhizomes commonly known as Tita roots constitute the drug. It is a tonic, stomachic and efficaceous in debility; also used in intermittent fevers.

Its active principles are alkaloids of the Berberine group. The drug has export value. Due to heavy exploitation, the natural population has become threatened and the export of the drug is restricted.

Species of *Thalictrum* and *Picrorhiza* are the main adulterants of this drug.

COSCINIUM[50]

Coscinium Fenestratum (Gaertn). Colebr.

Family : Menispermaceae.

Indian names : Hindi-*Jharihaldi.*

Description : A robust woody climbing shrub, bark yellowish, densely hairy when young; leaves leathery, shining, smooth on upper surface, slightly hairy on lower surface, roundish, with tapering tip, main nerves 5-7. Flowers minute, in small heads.

Distribution : The plant occurs in South India, chiefly in Western Ghats.

Drug and its Properties : The dried stems of the plant constitute the drug, the stems contain Berberine.

This drug is useful in fevers, general weakness or debility and certain types of dyspepsia. It is also considered antiseptic and is therefore, used for external application on wounds.

Roots of the plant are reported to show antibiotic activity.

Others Uses : The stems yield a yellow dye which is used singly or in combination with turmeric.

COSTUS[51]

Costus Speciosus (Koen, ex Retz.) Sm.

Family : Zingiberaceae.

Indian names : Hindi-*Keu.*

Description : An erect herb with rhizomatous horizontal root-stock. Leaves 15-30 cm long, almost without petiole, silky pubescent beneath. Flowers white with red bracts, tubular, in dense 5-13 cm long spike. Fruit red, trigonous (2 cm diameter) capsule; seeds black.

Distribution : This plant is fuound all over India, specially in plains and up to about 1,200 m; quite common in waste and user lands. It is also cultivated for ornament and for its rhizomes.

Drug and its Properties : The drug comprises the fresh and dried rhizomes of this plant. The rhizome is mucilaginous and feebly astringent. It is credited with purgative and tonic properties. The root is said to be depurgative and is used in Uttar Pradesh as a tonic, anthelmintic and aphrodisiac. Root is also used in catarrhal fever, cough, dyspepsia, worms, skin diseases and snake-bites.

This species is one of the indigenous sources for steroid synthesis; however, the percentage of diosgenin is lesser than in *Dioscorea* species.

Antifertility, antiinflammatory and anti-arthritic activity of steroidal compound isolated from this plant have beenexperimentally demonstrated. Some steroidal compounds have also shown local anaesthetic action.

Alkaloids from rhizomes have been found to possess antispasmodic, cardiotonic, hydrocholeratic and diuretic activities; also depressant on central nervous system.

Other Uses : The rhizome is edible after cooking. It is rich in starch, but the fibrous content is high in comparison to other tuberous food.

CYMBOPOGON[52]

Cymbopogon species.

Family : Poaceae.

Several species of the genus *Cymbopogon* grown in India, some are cultivated. Though medicinal properties have been attributed to some of these species, none of them is of much importance.

Grasses of the genus *Cymbopogon* are usually tall herbs and are aromatic. They yield oils which are largely used as flvouring agents. The important ones in this respect and in medicine are the following :

Cymbopogon citratus (CD.) Stapf is grown in several parts of India. It yields an oil called West India lemon-grass oil. An infusion of its leaves is sometimes taken as a substitute for tea, as a refershing beverage.

C. flexusous (Nees ex Steud.) Watson occurs in South India, Uttar Pradesh and Sikkim. It yields lemon-grass oil. This oil is source of Vatamin A. There are plantations of this grass in Kerala. It is also used in perfumery.

C. martinii (Roxb.) Watson (Hindi-*Rosha, Roshisha, Mirciagandh, Gandhvel)* occurs rather in all drier regions of India; it yields the Rosha oil which is useful on lumbago, baldness and on skin diseases; it is taken internally in bilicus complaints. This oil is also used for mosquito repellent ointments.

C. nardus (L.) Rendle grown in several parts of India, chiefly South India. It yields the well-known Citronella oil, which is used (like Rosha oil) in insect repellent ointments.

DATURA[53]

Datura stramonium L.

Family : Solanaceae.

Indian names : Hindi-*Dhatura.*

The trade names *Datura* and *Stramonium* are based on the scientific name of the plant. In old Inidan literature, the plant is referred as 'Shivashekhara', because the flower is believed to be associated with Lord Shiva.

Description : A bushy plant up to about 1 m high; leaves large, ovate, toothed. Flowers very large, white. Fruit ovoid deeply divided into four, covered with long or short prickles.

Distribution : The plant occurs in temperate Himalayas up ot 2,500 m and in hilly regions of central and southern India.

Drug and its Properties : The drug consists of dried leaves, flowering tops and seeds of the plant.

The chief active principle in the leaves is hyoscyamine; the drug is, therefore, useful in the same manner as *Belladonna* or *Hyoscyamus.* The drug is useful in bronchitis or asthma, and controls salivation in mouth; it is antispasmodic and narcotic. The inhalation of smoke from the burning leaves in also good for relieving asthma. The seeds also contain hyoscyamine and have similar properties as the leaves.

Other Species : Two other species of the genus *Datura* and useful in medicine.

D. metel L. occurs throughout India in waste places. Its flowers are white to yellowish, often violet coloured outside. Fruits have short prickles. In cultivation, the flowers often have double corolla whorls.

A poultice of its leaves checks inflammation of breasts caused by excssive formation of milk. The leaves and seeds have similar properties as *Stamonium.*

D. innoxia Mill. (Mar. Dhotra) is an exotic plant, but has run wild in several parts of India. The corolla of its flowers is 10-angled (not 5-angled as in *D. metel).* Fruits have very slender prickles and brown seeds. Its leaves have similar properties as *Stramonium.* Expansion of this plant through cultivation has been recommended.

DIGITALIS[54]

(Foxlove)

Digtalis Purpurea L.

Family : Scrophulariaceae.

Indian names : Hindi-*Tilpushpi.*

The trade name refers to the scientific aname of the plant. The Hindi name *Tipushpi* refers to the flowers of the plant which somewhat resemble the flowers of *Til* plant, *Sesamum indicum* L.

Description : A biennial or perennial herb up to about 1.2 m high; lower basal leaves long-stalked, hairy, ovate, 15-30 cm long, the upper leaves almost without stalks, becoming smaller in size upwards. Flowers 5-8 cm long, white or purple, with ciliate lobes, borne in 30-60 cm long, one-sided bunches. Fruit ovoid.

Distribution : This plant is not indigeneous to India, it is cultivated chiefly in hilly regions of northern India, such as in Kashmir; it was grown in Darjeeling and in Nilgiri hills also but these cultivations are now abandoned. The plants have ascaped from cultivation and have become naturalised in some places.

Drug and its Properties : The dried leaves of the plant constitute the drug. The leaves must be dried at about 60°C temperature and as soon as possible after collection.

The main use of this drug is in heart diseases. The drug promotes and stimulates the activity of all muscle tissue. It is used in cases of congested heart failure.

Digitalis forces more blood into the coronaries and improves the nutrition of the heart. When blood circulation gets impaired and dropsy sets in, *Digitalis* helps in restoration and regulation of the function of the heart.

It improves the blood supply to the kideny and this promotes urination, and removes obstructions in kidney.

Digitalis is used in some. ointments for local application on wounds and burns. This drug, however, has some cumulative toxic effects and causes headache, giddiness, etc. These side-effects must be watched.

Other Species : Another species of the genus *Digitalis,* viz. *D. lanata* Ehrh. (Woolly Foxglove), is being cultivated and also occurs as ascape in Kashmir. Its flowers are smaller, hiry, and cream-yellow, or purple-coloured. This plant has stronger medicinal properties, and its side-effects are not so toxic as of *D.purpurea.*

DIOSCOREA[55]

Dioscorea species.

Family : Dioscoreaceae.

This is a large genus of twining herbs. In some species the stems twine to the right, and in others to the left. Leaves are simple or compound; mostly the nerves are prominent. The tubers in most species have tuberous roots, and also tuber-like round or variously shaped structure (bulbils) in axil of leaves.

About 50 species are found in India; several are cultivated for edible tubers, the Yams.

The genus has recently gained much repute as a source fo steroidal sapogenins, like diosgenin. These are promising strting material for synthesis of cortisone; which is useful in treatment of reheumatic arthritis, and in preparation of sex hormones.

Dioscorea deltoidea Wall. (Punjab-*Kriss, Kitra;* Kashmir- *Kins, Kithi Kildri)* is an extensive climeber occurring in north-western Himalayas, and extending to central Himalayas. Its tubers are rich in diosgenin.

D. prazeri Prain and Burkill (syn. *D. deltoidea* Wall. var. *sikkimensis* Prain, D. *sikkimensis* Prain and Burkill) occurs in eastern Himalayas, in northern parts of Bihar, Bengal, Nepal,

Sikkim, Bhutan and Assam. It has now been successfully grown in other parts of India. The tubers are rich in diosgenin.

Other Uses Yams are a common article of food particularly among the hill tribes and the poor.

D. alata L. (Hindi and Benagli-*Khamalu, Chuprialu;* Kanarese-*Onthalaigasu, Tung-genasu;* Malayalam-*Kaavathu;* Tamil-*Perumvallikizhongu;* Telugu-*Pendalamu)* is a large climber and is grown for its edible tubers. *D. bulvifera* L., *D. hipida* Dennst. and *D. Pentaphylla* L. occur almost throughout India; their tubers are also edible, and are consumed after proper processing.

Some species of *Dioscorea* yield industrial starch.

CARDAMOM[56]

Elettaria Cardamomum (L) Maton.

Family : Zingiberaceae.

Indian names : Hindi-*Chhoti Ilaichi.*

Description : A herb with thick, fleshy branched rhizome and several erect stems, going sometimes up to 3 m high. Leaves very large, 30-90 cm long, narrow, with one strong median nerve and numerous faint side nerves. Flowering stock arises near the base of the stem and lies on the ground; flowers about 4 cm long, white or pale green, borne in 30-90 cm long bunches. Fruits about 1.5 cm long, pale green to yellow, ovoid; 3-celled, many-seeded. Seeds triangular, brownish-black. The size of the plant and of its parts varies in different localities and with different cultivated races. The fruits and seeds, however, do not vary much. Often, the fruits offered in market are bleached with sulphur fumes and made white.

Distribution : It occurs wild in southern India, particularly in the moist forests of hilly regions in mysore and Kerala. It is also cultivated elsewhere in India.

Drug and its Properties : The dried fruits of the plant constitute the drug. The seeds are actually used, but they are taken out from the fruits just when required.

Cardamom is used chiefly for relieving flatulence or feeling of overfullness of stomach, i.e. to promote digestion. It is administered with purgatives, and as a flavouring agent. Powdered with cloves, ginger and caraeway, it is good in indigestion, etc.

Other Uses : *Cardamoms* are largely used in cooking and in making cakes and confectionery. The oil obtained from seeds is used for flavouring beverages.

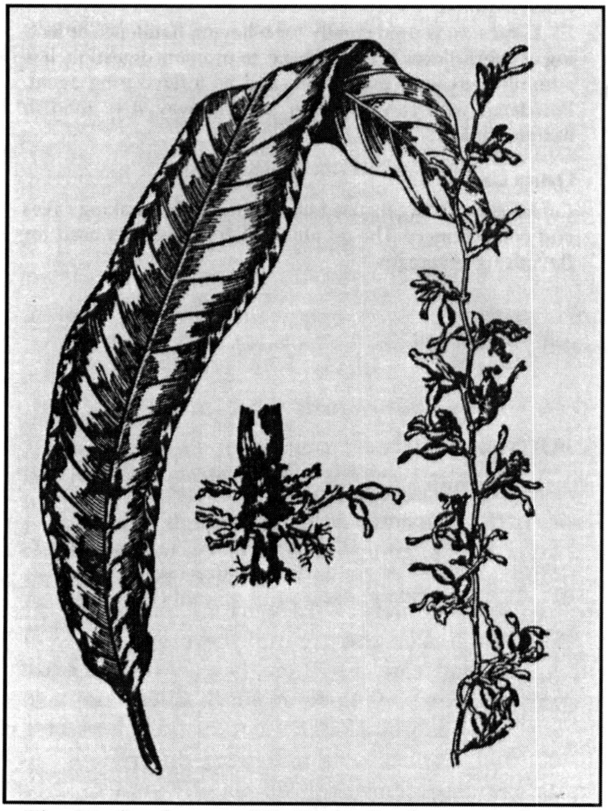

Fig. 10. Cardamom (Elettaria Cardamomum).

EMBELIA[57]

Embelia Tsjeriam-Cottam A. D.C. = *E. acutipetalum* (Lam. ex tlassk.) Almeida and Almeida.

Family : Mayrsinaceae.

Indian names : Hindi-*Baibirang, Bhungi, Gaiya.*

The trade name is based on the scientific name of the plant.

Description : A shrub or small tree; young branches covered with brownish hairs, mature branches glabrous; braches specked with white glands. Leaves up to 12 cm long, narrowed at bouth ends, dotted all over with glands, margins simpler or toothed, leaves sometiems reddish on lower surface, hairy on nerves. Flowers minute, pale green, in short, axillary, densely hairy clusters. Fruit small, globose, pointed, red when ripe.

Distribution : This plant occurs chiefly in eastern India and the Deccan peninsula.

Drug and its Properties : The dried fruit of the plant constitutes the drug. The main use of this drug is in treatment of tapeworms. Given in suitable doses, the drug kills the tapeworms; they are then expelled with the help of a purgative. *Embelia* itself has mild laxative property. Recent experiments have shown that the drug is effective only against tapeworms not hookworms and roundworms. It also destroys earthworms and should be useful in ascariasis. The drug also showed some antibacterial and antitubercular activity.

Other Species : An allied species, *Embelia ribes* Burm. f., is found throughout India. This plant is also known generally by same local names as *E. tsjeriam-cottam*. Its fruits have similar properties too, and are also accepted to constitute the official drug *Embelia.*

EMBLICA[58]

(Emblic Myrobalan)

Emblica Officinalis Gaertn.=*Phyllanthus emblica* L.

Family : Euphorbiaceae

Indian names : Hindi-*Aonla.*

The trade name *Emblica* is based on the scientific name. It is also called *Emblic Myrobalan* as it is one of the three well-known Myrobalans.

Destcription : A small or middle-sized deciduous tree. Leaves small, 10-13 mm long, 2-3 mm broad, very closely set in pinnate fashion, branchlets look rather feathery in general appearance. Male and female flowers borne on same tree, flowers pale green, usually in small dense clusters below the leaves; male flowers small, numerous, on short stalks; female flowers also small, fewer. Fruit 1.5-2.5 cm diameter, fleshy, roundish, rather indistinctly marked into 6 lobes, pale green or yellowish; seeds 6. Fruits of cultivated farms are larger.

Distribution : The plant occurs throughout tropical and sub-tropical India; it was found to be abundant (and practially unexploited) in deciduous forests of Madhya Pradesh.

Drug and its Properties : The fresh or dried fruits of this tree constitute the drug.

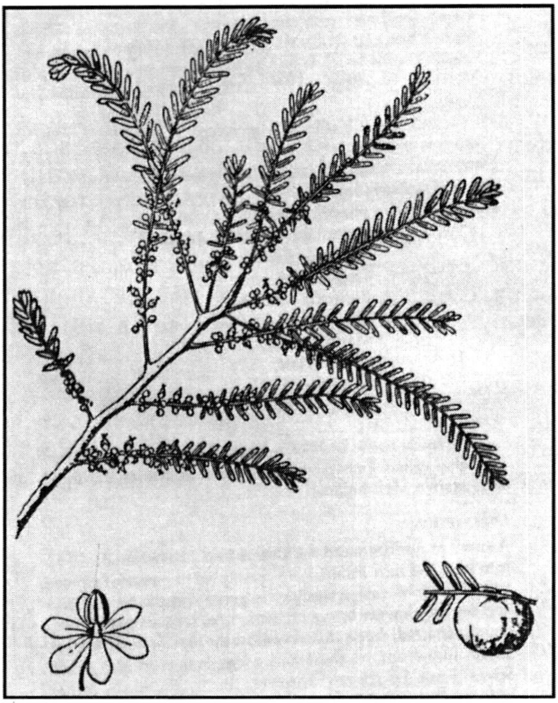

Fig. 11. Emblica (Emblic Myrobalan).

The fruits are one of the three constituents of the well-known Indian preparation *Triphala* (the other two constitutents being *Bahera-Terminalia bellirica* -and *Harra-T. chebula). Triphala* is used as laxative and in treatment of enlarged liver, piles, stomach complaints, pain in eyes, etc.

Emblica fruits are a good liver tonic; raw fruits are cooling and mild laxative. A fermented liquor made from the fruits is considered useful in indigestion, anaemia, jaundice, certain heart complaints, cold in nose and for promoting urination. It is a very rich source of vitamin C, and is valuable in diseases caused by deficiency of vitamin C, like scurvy. Certain experiments on patients of pulmonary tuberculosis showed that vitamin C of *Emblica* fruits is more quickly assimilated in human system than synthetic vitamin C; perhaps there are certain unknown factors in the fruits responsible for this advantage. Dried fruits are useful in diarrhoea and dysentery. Even pickled fruits are prescribed in Indian medicine.

Flowers, roots and bark of the tree are also medicinal, seeds are reported to cure asthma and stomach disorders.

Other uses : Fruits are largely used in inks and dyes and for hair shampoos; fruits along with twig bark are employed for tanning and dyeing.

The timber is useful for miscellaneous domestic purposes; it stands well under water and is used in making wells etc.

Leaves are used as manure in *Cardamom* plantations; they also help in improvement of alkali soils.

EPHEDAR[59]

Ephedra Gerardiana Wallich.

Family : Gnetaceae.

Indian names : Hindi-*Asmania, Phok, Khanda.*

The trade name is based on the scientific name.

Description : A small shrub up to about 1 m high. Stems woody below, much branched; branches almost whorled, erect or initially a little spreading and then ascending upwards. Leaves reduced to minute 2-toothed sheaths. Male flowers few together in ovate spikes. Female flowers 1-2, in short spikes. Fruits 7-10 mm long, ovoid, red, surrounded by succulent bracts.

Distribution : This plant occurs in the drier regions of higher Himalayan ranges, at about 2,000-4,000 m. It is also cultivated.

Drug and its Properties : The dried stems of *Ephedra gerardiana,* collected in autumn, constitute the drug *Ephedra.*

The main use of this drug, which yields Ephedrine, is in treatment of asthma, particularly bronchial asthma. For relieving bronchial spasms, the drug is administered orally or through injections. The drug is useful as a stimulant for heart. In cases where heart is affected by infections of pneumonia, diphtheria, etc. *Ephedra* proves a very effective cardiac stimulant.

It has also been used in hay-fever, rashes, etc., of allergic origin. Several preparations based on Ephedrine are in use in medicine nowadays. Nasal sprays are used in sinusitis, asthmatic attacks, inflammation of mucous membrane, etc.

As the drug has some effect on the urinary bladders also, it is used to control night wetting (urinating while sleeping) in children.

Overdoses of Ephedrine can cause nausea, sweating, certain skin diseases, etc.

Other Species : Another species of the genus *Ephedra,* namely *E. major* Host, occurs in Lahul; it has more alkaloids than *E. gerardiana,* and branches of both these species, are therefore, accepted as the drug *Ephedra.*

Regular supplies of the drug can be ascertained only if these two plants, or the Chinese species, *E. equisetina* Bunge and *E. Sinica* Stapf, which are better sources of Ephedrine, are cultivated.

Several areas in northern Himalayas, such as higher altitudes in Kashmir, Punjab, Himachal Pradesh and Uttar pradesh, are suitable for cultivation of *Ephedra* species.

EUPHORBIA[60]

Euphorbia Hirta L. syn. *E. piluifera* (of Indian floras, not of Linneaus).

Family : Euphorbiaceae.

Indian names : Hindi-*Lal Dudhi.*

The trade name is based on the scientific name of the plant.

Description : An annual herb ascending or erect up to 50 cm high; stems round, covered with yellowish hairs. Leaves in opposite pairs, small, up to about 4 cm long, dark green on upper side, pale on lower side, margins faintly toothed. Flowers whitish, minute, in small, axillry, stalked clusters. Fruit small, 1-2 mm diameter, hairy; seeds 3-angled, wrinkled, light reddish brown.

Distribution : The plant occurs in waste place throughout the warmer regions of India, and in a variety of soil and moisture conditions.

Drug and its Properties : The entire plant, collected in flowering and fruiting stage and dried, constitutes the drug.

Euphorbia causes relaxation of bronchioles, and has a depressant action on heart and respiration. It is useful in removing worms in children, in bowel complaints, asthma and cough. The plant promotes formation and flow of milk in women; it is also useful in gonorrhoea and other urinogenital complaints. The roots of the plant stop vomiting, Large doses of the drug, however, cause irritation in stomach and resrult in vomiting and nausea.

The milky juice of the plant is applied on warts. The antibacterial and antitubercular activity of the plant has been shown experimentally.

Other Uses : The leaves of *Euphorbia hirta* are eaten as vegetable.

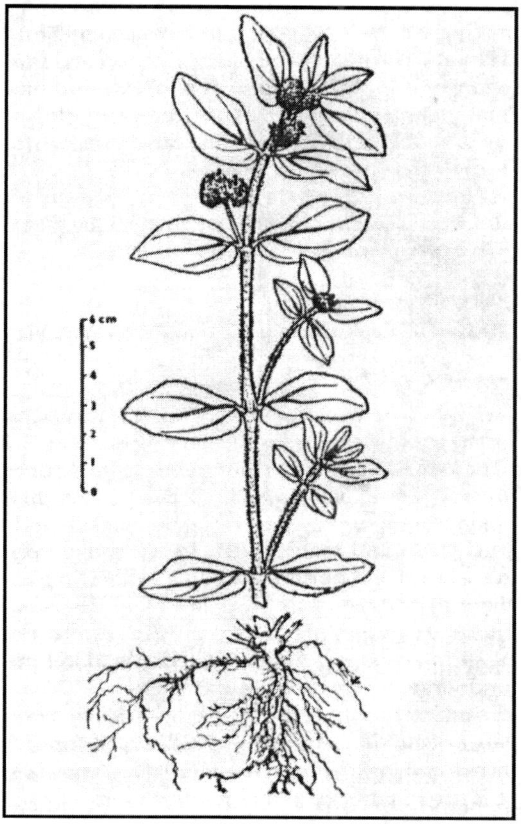

Fig. 12. Euphorbia (Euphorbia Hirta).

Other Species : A few other herbaceous species of the genus have been reported to have similar medicianl properties as *E. hirta.*

The genus *Euphorbia* includes some large shrubby species easily recognised by their thick, succulent, very throny (Cactus-like) round or characteristically angled and spirally twisted stems and branches. The white milky juice of such plants is acrid and pooisonous. Careless handling of the juice of these plants can cause skin and other diseases. Only in restricted doses they are used as purgatives, etc. The juice of some of the species is applied externally to kill maggots in wounds and on skin diseases and warts.

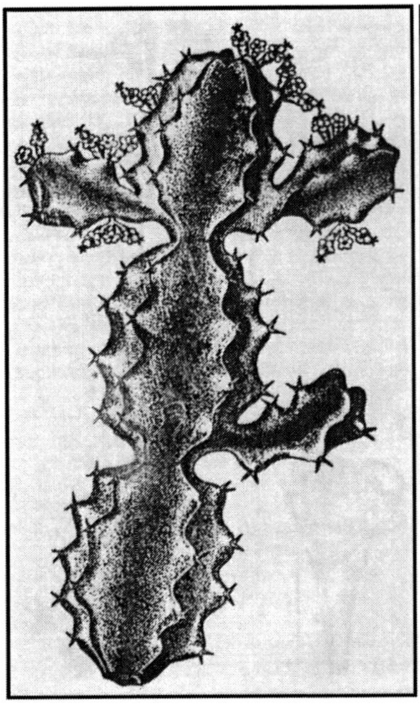

Fig. 13. Euphorbia (Euphorbia antiquorum).

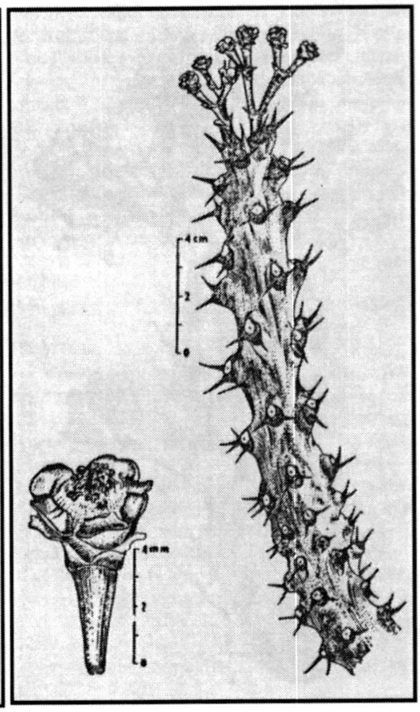

Fig. 14. Euphorbia (Euphorbia neriifolia).

E. antiquorum L. (Fig 13 Hindi-*Tridhari Sehund,* Kannada-*Kedaravalli,* Sanskrit-*Vajrakantaka)* has 3-5 angled branches and grows throughout India in warmer regions. Its juice is usedin dropsy and as nervine tonic.

E. barnhartii Croizat syn. *E. trigona* Roxb. (Telugu-*Kattimandu)* occurs in dry rocky hills of Deccan and in Andamans. Powdered leaves are used as poultice on boils.

Picture place

E. neriifolia L. (Fig. 14 Hindi-*Sehund, Thuhar;* Sanskrit- *Snuhi)* has 5-angled branches; it grows wild in Deccan peninsula, but is cultivated in hedges throughout India. Its juice is used in earache and asthma.

E. nivulia Buch.- Ham. (Hindi-*Katathuhar,* Sanskrit-*Patrasnuhi)* has cylindrical branches and occurs almost throughout India in drier regions. This too is grown in hedges. Its juice is believed to be diuretic.

(The tribals of Bastar use the white juice for treating wounds of cattle).

E. royleana Boiss. (Punjabi-*Danda Thor*) has 5-7 angled banches and occurs on outer dry slopes of western Himalayas, usually between 1,000-1,500 m altitude.

E. tirucalli L. (Hindi-*Sehund,* Kannada-*Kolukalli,* Sanskrit-*Vajradruma*) is a shrub or small tree with muchbranched cylindric branches; branches much narrower than other species. It is an African species but largely planted in hedges and on roadsides throughout drier parts of India, chiefly in Deccan and western India. The white juice of the plant is considered useful for local application in rheumatic pains, toothache, etc. In small doses, it is also given internally.

ASAFOETIDA[61]

Ferula Narthex Boiss.

Family : Apiaceae.

Indian names : Hindi–*Hing.*

The trade name is based on the scientific name of a related species *Ferula assafoetida* L., which yields similar drug.

Description : A tall perennial herb with robust carrot-shaped roots. Leaves of two kinds; lower simple, 30-60 cm. long, ovate; upper much divided into numerous segments. Yound leaves densely hairy. Flowers small, yellow, in large terminal clusters, Fruit 8 mm long, about half as broad or broader.

Distribution : This plant grows in Kashmir.

Drug and its Properties : *Asafoetida* is the resinous and scented substance obtained by incision n the lliving rhizomes or roots of this plant and its allied species.

It is a very useful remedy for relieving spasms and indigestion, flatulent colic, cholera and whooping cough. It is a stimulant for respiratory and nervous system and is very effective in pneumonia and bronchitis in children. It is applied externally on stomach to stimulalte the intestines, even its enema is recommended in intestinal flatulence.

Experiments have shown that *Asafoetida* has some sedative properties and its possible use in heart disease has been suggested.

Other Uses : *Asafoetida* is largely used as a spice; it is an essential ingredient in most pulses and vegetable curry preparations, pickles, etc.

Other Species : Several species of this genus occuring in Central Asian region (A fghanistan, etc.) such as *F. foetida* (Bung) Regel and *F. assafoetida* L. yield similar products as *F. narthex.*

WINTERGREEN[62]

Gaultheria Fragrantissima Wallich.

Family : Ericaceae.

Indian Names: Hindi–*Gandhpura-ka-tel.*

The trade name is based on the volatile oil, called *Wintergreen Oil,* obtained from this plant.

Description : An evergreen shrub about 3 m high. Stems much-branched, bark orange-brown. Leaves up to 13 cm. long, rather broad, leathery, dotted with glands, margins toothed. Flowers small, greenish white, in short axillary bunches. Fruit roundish, enclosed in blue sepals.

Distribution : This plant occurs in the hilly regions of northern, eastern and southern India, between 1,500 and 2,500 m altitude.

Drug and its Properties : The *Wintergreen Oil* is the volatile oil obtained from fresh plants of this species.

This oil is used in treatment of various forms of rheumatism. It is applied locally; it is also added to certain ointments and liniments to counteract their irritating effects. It is useful in destroying hookworms and also has stimulant and carminative properties.

It is interesting to mention that when small qunatities of this oil are administered to experimental mice, development of cancer is delayed. The drug has also prevented or cured certain types of tumor formation in animals.

Other Uses : The oils is used as a flavouring agent in soft drinks, lemon drops, toothpastes, etc. The oil is also used in many preparations for killing or repelling mosquitoes, files and other insects. The plant is grown as an ornament in hill stations of India.

INDIAN GENTIAN[63]

Gentiana Kurroo Royle

Family : Gentianaceae.

Indian names : Hindi–*Kamalphul, Kutki, Nilkanth.*

The trade name indicates that it is the Indian substitute of true *Gentian*.

Description : A small perennial herb with tufted decumbent stems, 10-30 cm high. Rootstock thick. Lower basal leaves 7-13 cm long, tufted; upper leaves up to 2.5 cm long, narrow. Flowers blue, with white spots, 4.5 cm long, 2-2.5 cm diameter, arising singly or in small bunches or 2-4 flowers. Fruit about 2 cm long.

Distribution : This plant occurs in north-western Himalayas, between 1,300 and 3,500 m altitude, in Kashmir and adjoining hills.

Drug and its Properties : This dried rhizomes of the plant constitute the drug.

Gentian is used for improving appetite and stimulating gastric secretion. It is an ingredient of many tonic and stomachic preparations. It has pleasant flavour and is afreeable to taste. In causes purging.

Other Species *: Gentiana lutea* L. (Yellow Gentian) is a foreign species, its roots are much valued in medicine and are largely imported into India. It has been suggested that the climate of northwestern Himalayas at altitudes of about 3,000 m should be suitable for its cultivation.

One or two more species of *Gentiana* occur wild in the Himalayas; they can also be used as substitute for *Gentiana kurroo.*

An Indian plant *Picrorhiza kurrooa* is considered suitable substitute for *G. lutea.*

LIQUORICE[64]

Glycyrrhiza Glabra L.

Family : Fabaceae.

Indian names : Hindi–*Mulahti, Mulethi.*

The trade name *Liquorice* should not be mixed with the drug called *Indian Liquorice,* Which comes from an entirely different plant *Abrus precatorius* L. (Gunja).

Description : A tall erect herb or undershrub up to about 1.5 m high. Leaves compound, leaflets 4-7 pairs. Flowers lilac or light violet, small, in slender axillary spikes which are equal to, or slightly longer than the leaves. Fruits 1-3 cm long, flat, densely covered all over with small spinous outgrowths. The rootstock throws numerous additional roots, or in some forms, there are several branched stems near the rootstock remaining underground.

Distribution : The plant is being underground stems of this plant constitute the drug.

Liquorice is believed to be useful in cough, sore throat, bronchitis, abdominal pains, consumption and epilepsy. For sorethroat and cough, a small piece of raw *Liqorice* is just chewed or sucked.

Liquorice promotes urination, and its diuretic activity, as also antibiotic and antibacterial activity, have been experimentally shown.

Due to its sweet taste and demulcent property, *Liquorice* is largely used in making syrups and for masking bitter taste of medicines in mixtures or pills; it is useful in gastric and duodenal ulcers.

Liquorice power, mixed with butter (ghee) and honey, is applied on cuts and wounds.

The leaves of the plant, if applied as a poultice, are believed to be useful in scalds of the hands.

Other Uses : The powder or small pieces of the drug are commonly taken with betel leaves *(Pan).*

Kashmir, Punjab, Himachal Pradesh, Uttar Pradesh and Madras have been suggested as suitable areas for cultivation of this plant.

During a discussion on this plant, the late Dr. H. Santapau, Director, Botanical Survey of India (who was born in Spain and later became an Indian national) recalled that *Glycyrrhiza* is a very widespread weed in rice fields in Spain and Italy. Yound boys would rather pick up fresh pieces of its roots and suck, than buy toffees.

INDIAN SARSAPARILLA[65]

(Hemidesmus, Anantmul)

Hemidesmusindicus (L) Schult.

Family : Periplocaceae.

Indian names : Hindi–*Anantmul, Salsa.*

As the drug obtained from this plant serves as substitute for the true *Sarsaparilla* (which is the product of the genus *Smilax*), it is called *Indian Sarssaparilla.*

Description : A perennial twiner or creeper, rootstock woody, fragrant; stems slender, hairless; leaves very greatly in shape and size, they are 5-10 cm long, but their breadth varies from 5 to about 4 cm, dark green, often with whitish blotches, pale or whitish, hairy on lower furface. Flowers very small, greenish, in small, compact cluster. Fruits 10-15 cm long, green, narrow, cylindric, pointed at tip, in pairs. Seeds small, black, with a tuft of white hairs at top, all parts of the plant have white milky juice.

Distribution : The plant occurs almost throughout India.

Drug and its Properties : The dried roots of the plants constitute the drug.

The drug is useful in fever, skin diseases, loss of appetite, syphilis, leucorrhoea and other urinary complaints. The diuretic action of the drug has been shown experimentally. The drug is largely used as a blood purifier and in rheumatism. Tests in hospitals have confirmed the utility of *Indian Sarsaparilla* as a substitute for true *Sarsaparilla,* which is obtained from plants of the genus *Smilax.*

Other Uses : The leaves of the narrow-leaved form of the plant are chewed and are refreshing.

KURCHI[66]

Holarrhena Antidysenterica (Roth) A. DC.

Family : Apocynaceae.

Indian names : Hindi–*Indrajau, Korai, Kurchi.*

The trade name is based on the local Indian name of the plant; the word *antidysenterica* in the scientific name indicates its chief usage. The Sanskrit name 'Kutaja' denotes, it grows on peaks (*Kut : peak).*

Description : A tall shrub or small tree, sometimes up to m tall. Leaves 10-30 cm long, ovate, thin, nerves on the leaves conspicuous. Leafstalks very small. Flowers white, fragrant, 1-1.5 cm diameter, in large terminal bunches. Fruits slender, cylindric, 20-45 cm long, 6-8 mm thick, dark grey with white specks all over. Seeds about 1 cm long, having a tuft of long (2-2.5 cm) brown hairs at top. All parts of the plant, on incision, give out white milky juice.

Distribution : The plant occurs througout India up to an altitude of about 1,200 m. It was found to be very common on forest fringes in Madhya Pradesh and Maharashtra.

Drug and its Properties : The dried bark of the plant constitutes the drug *kurchi.*

The chief use of this drug is in amoebic dysentery. Either an extract of the bark is used singly or several other preparations in combination with chemical compounds are used. The bark of the plant also has tonic and febrifuge properties.

The alkaloid Conessine present in this bark has been found to retard growth of tubercular bacillii.

Seeds also possess alkaloids which are effective in dysentery.

Certain madicinal properties have been attributed to leaves also.

Other Uses : This plant is good for afforestation of poor soils; it is a pioneer in newly cleared forest areas. The wood is good for making miscellaneous domestic articles such as paper knives, toys, small boxes, pen holders, printing blocks, tobacco pouches, picture frames, etc.

CHALMOGRA[67]

Hydnocarpus Kurzii (King) Warb.

Family : Flacourtiaceae.

Indian names : Hindi–*Chalmogra.*

Description : A tree about 15 m high, sometimes more, with a tall trunk and a crown of drooping branches. Leaves about 20 cm long, pointed at tip, leathery. Flowers small, yellow, in small axillary clusters. Fruit 6-7 cm diameter, round, brown; seeds many.

Distribution : The tree is found in evergreen forests of Assam and Tripura; at certain spots it is very aboundant.

Drug and its Properties : The oil obtained from the fresh ripe seeds of the tree is medicinal.

The oil is used in treatment of leprosy. Formerly the oil was given orally, now certain preparations based on the oil are injected. The bark of the tree contains certain tannins and is considered useful in fever.

Other Uses : The seed-cake of *Hydnocarpus kurzii* as manure. Some animals eat the fruits of this tree; it has been recommended that the flesh of such animals should not be eaten. Even fish stupefied or killed by *Chalmogra* fruits are considered unsuitable for human consumption.

Other Species : *Hydnocarpus laurifolia* (Dennst) Sleummer syn. *H. wightiana* Blume (Marathi–*Katukavath,* Sanskrit–*Garuphal,* Tamil–*Maravetti)* occurs in the Western Ghats. The oil from the seeds is medicinal. Its has similar properties as the oil from. H. *Kurzii.* It is applied locally on leprosy and reduces the nodules. The oil is useful also on rheumatic pains, sprains, tubercular laryngitis, inflammations, etc. Some experiments have shown its effect in destroying certain bacteria.

TALMAKHANA[68]

Hygrophila Auriculata (Schum) Heine.

Syn. *H. spinosa* and., *Asteracantha longifolia* Nees.

Family : Acanthaceae.

Indian names : Hindi–*Kuliakanta, Talmakhana*

Description : A stout erect herb, 60-150 cm high; stems unbranched, erect, straight, four-angled, hairy, more so below the swollen nodes. Leaves whorled, 6 at a node, each having a sharp, yellow spine in its axil. Flowers 8 in a whorl, purple-blue, about 3 cm long, 2-lipped; lower lip characteristically folded.

Distribution : The plant occurs in marshes and other moist spots throughout India, often the shallow, partially dried ditches and roadside water channels.

Drug and its properties : The drug consists of the entire plant including the roots.

It is useful in dropsy, jaundice, rheumatism and disease of urinogenital system; seeds are considered useful also in venereal diseases. The diuretic activity of the drug is believed to be due to combination of both inorganic and organic contents of the plants. Seeds and roots, singly also, have diuretic property. Leaves are useful in cough and urethral discharges.

HYOSCYAMUS[69]

(*Indian Henbane*)

Hyoscyamus Niger L. Plate II.

Family : Solanaceae.

Indian names : Hindi–*Khurasani Ajvain.*

Description : An annual or biennial bad-smelling herb, densely covered with glandular hairs; stem up to 1 m high. Lower basal leaves 15-20 cm, margins toothed. Upper leaves smaller and divided into many segments. Flowers 2-3 cm diameter, pale green, streaked with purple, some borne solitary at the place of branching of stems, others in long, terminal spikes, Fruits 1.3 cm diameter, globose.

Distribution : The plant occurs in the western Himalayas from Kashmir to Garhwal at altitudes of about 1,500 m to 3,000 m, commonly in waste places near habitations. It has been cultivated in several regions of India, such as Kashmir, Punjab, Uttar Pradesh, maharashtra and Nilgiri hills.

Drug and its Properties : The dried leaves and flowering tops collected soon after flowering of the plant constitute the drug.

The drug has similar properties as *Belladnna (Atropa belladonna).* It is useful for relieving certain painful spasmodic conditions of muscles, and in hysteria, cough, etc. It also dilates the pupil of the eye.

Seeds of the plant also have medicinal properties, they are usually, pasted and applied locally on pains.

It can be grown in the Himalayan region in Kashmir, Punjab, Himachal Pradesh and Uttar Pradesh.

Other Species : *Hyoscyamus muticus* L. *(Egyptian Henbane)* is being cultivated in Kashmir, etc. The alkaloic content of this plant is more than *Indian Henbane;* it also has more intense narcotic property. The leaves of *Egyptian Henbane* are smoked for intoxication.

KALADANA[70]

Ipomoea Nil (L.) Roth syn. *I. hederacea* auct. non Jacq.

Family : Convolvulaceae.

Indian names : Hindi–*Kaladana, Nikalmi.*

Description : An annual twining plant, stems sparsely covered with hairs. Leaves 5-12 cm diameter, ovate, shallowly or deeply 3-lobed. Flowers 4-5 cm long, funnel-shaped, blue, slightly orange-coloured below, few growing together in small stalked clusters. Fruit 8 mm diameter, almost roundish or ovoid. Seeds, small, glabrous. There is an interesting thing about colour of flowers. Flowers are blue as long as they are on the plants; within minutes of plucking they become purplish; this is why many books mention of flowers as purple.

Distribution : The plant occurs throughout India up to an altitude of about 1,800 m; it is truly wild in India; at times it is cultivated.

Drug and its Properties : The dried seeds of the plant constitute the drug cause irritation.

Kaladana is used as a purgative. Overdoses of the drug cause irritation.

Other Uses : Fresh fruits of the plant are eaten as vegetable. The plant is often grown for its beautiful flowers.

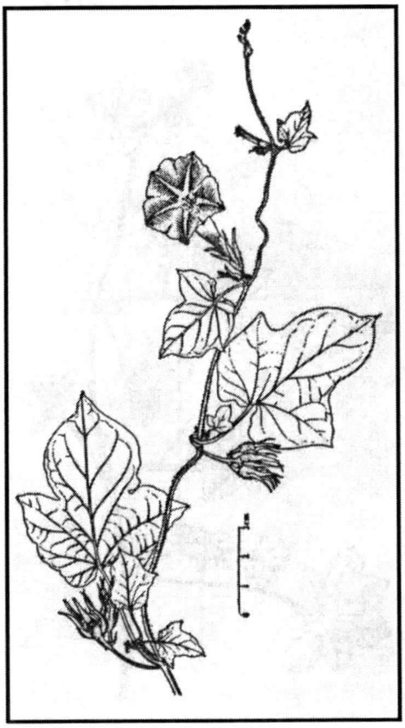

Fig. 15. Kaladana (Ipomoea Nil).

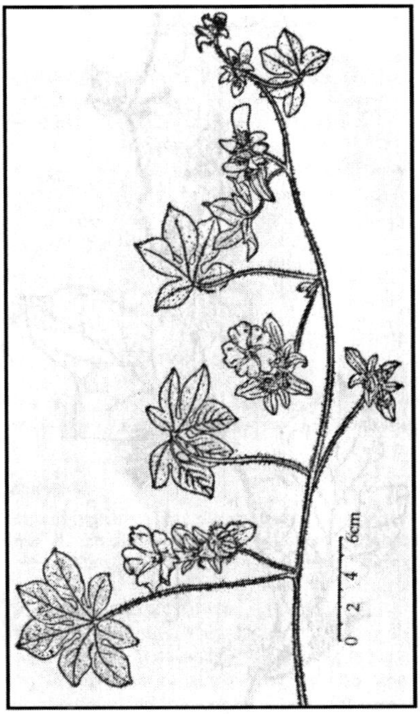

Fig. 16. Ipomoea pestigridis.

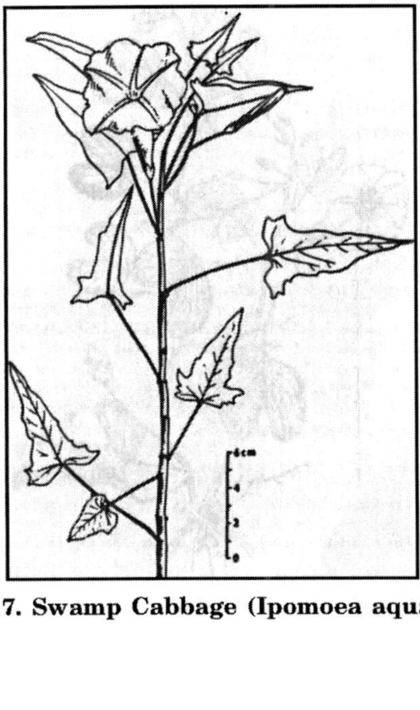

Fig. 17. Swamp Cabbage (Ipomoea aquatica).

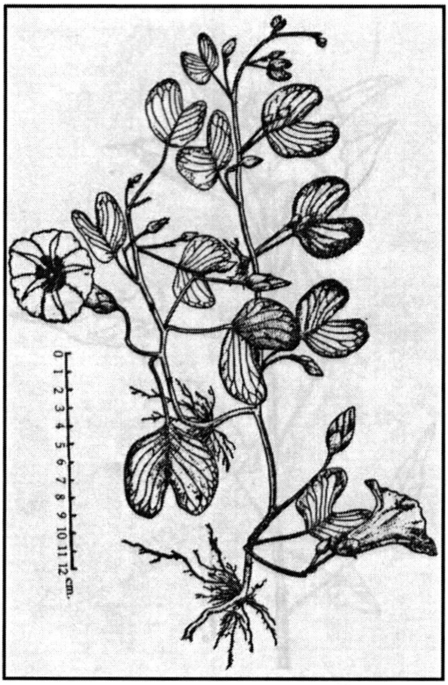

Fig. 18. Ipomoea (Ipomoea pescaprae).

Other Species : Several other species of the genus *Ipomoea* are of medicinal value. Many of them have laxative or purgative properties. For example, roots of *Ipomoea pestigridis* L. (Fig. 17 Hindi-*Ghiabati, Kaladana, Panchpatri,* Madhya Pradesh–*Badi Pasvi*) juice of whole plant of I. aquatica Forsk (Fig. 18 Swamp cabbage, Hindi–*Kalmishak,* Panjabi–*Sornalika-sag*), *I. pescaprae* (L) Roth (Morning glory), *I. quamoclit* L. (Indian Pink, Hindi–*Kamlata,* Bengali–*Torulata*) and *I. uniflora* Roem and Schult and seeds of *I. cairica* (L) Sweet (Railway Creeper) are considered to be laxative or purgative.

(The tribals of Bastar crush the flowers of *I. aquatica* and put the juice into inflammed eyes.)

The tuberous roots of *Ipomoea purga* Heyne (which is now named as *Exogonium purga* Benth) are laxative. this plant is a native of America; it has been cultivated in gardesn for ornament or otherwise, in several places particularly in southern and eastern India. Indian species are, however, its satisfactory substitutes.

HENNA[71]

LAWSONIA INERMIS L. syn. L. alba L.

Family : Lythraceae.

Indian names : Hindi – *Mehndi.*

Description : A Middle-sized or large, much-branched shrub, sometimes tree-like; branches 4-angled, usually ending in a sharp point. Leaves opposite, 2-3 cm long, often acute and sharp-pointed. Flowers small, white or pinkish, fragrant, in terminal large bunches. Fruit small, size of a pea, round; seeds many.

Distribution : The plant occurs in several parts of India, chiefly in the drier parts of the peninsula, but is usually cultivated in hedges. It is also cultivated for commerce in Punjab, Gujarat, Madhya Pradesh and Rajasthan.

Drug and its Properties : The leaves of the plant have certain medicinal properties.

They are astringent and are used as a prophylactic against skin diseases. They are applied locally on boils, burns and skin diseases. A decoction of leaves is used as gargle in sore throat. The paste of leaves is largely used in Indian homes in headache, burning sensation in feet, etc.

The leaves have also been shown to have some action against tubercular and other bacteria, and in typhoid and haemorrhagia. The plant has not, however, so far been put to much use in this manner.

Other Uses : The chief use of the *Henna* plant is as pleasant orange dye for colouring, palms, nails, feet, hair, beard, even tails and limbs of animals, *Henna,* mixed with other natural dyes, is largely used as hairdye and even for textiles.

The oil obtained from its flowers is used in perfumery.

LOBELIA[72]

(Wild tobacco)

Lobelia Nicotianaefolia Heyne ex Roth.

Family : Lobeliaceae.

Indian names *:* Hindi–*Narasal.*

Description : A large herb; stem stout, hollow, 3-5 m high, occasionally branched in the upper part. Leaves very large, up to 45 cm long in lower part of stem, smaller upwards, margins notentire; the main nerve of the leaves whitish. Flowers large, white, in very large terminal bunches. Fruit 8 mm, roundish. Seeds many, small, yellowish, brown.

Distribution : The plant occurs in the hilly regions of the Deccan peninsula, also in adjoining plains.

Drug and its Properties : The drug consists of aerial parts of the plant collected in October to November and dried in shade.

The properties of this drug are somewhat similar to nicotine. It is used in bronchitis and asthma; the drug causes sweating, nausea and consequently vomiting, thereby causing general relaxation. The drug is sometimes dangerous in the sense that if it is not vomited out, it is toxic to the system, and even death may occur.

Lobeline, the alkaloid contained in this drug, stimulates respiration and is used for reviving respiration in cases of failures of respiration caused by excessive narcotics, anesthesias, gases, etc.

Aerial parts of *L. nicotianaefolia* exude a white juice; this juice causes blisters on skin.

The dried plants seem to cause irritation of mucous membrance (such as in nose and throat) even from some distance. Coolies engaged for plant collection work avoid aproaching areas inhabited by this plant.

Other Species : *Lobelia inflata* is a plant of America and efforts are being made to cultivate it in India. Deccan Peninsula and Assam are considered to be better areas for its cultivation. The drug *Lobelia,* which yields Lobeline, is imported into India. However, *lobelia* drug obtained from Indian species described above is used as substitute.

A few other less important species of *Lobelia* grow wild in India but are not of much use.

MADHUCA[73]

Madhuca indica Gmel. syn. Bassia latifolia Roxb.

Family : Sapotaceae.

Indian names : Hindi–*Mahua, Mahuva.*

Description : A large deciduous tree with rather shorter bole, but larger crown. Leaves 12-25 cm long, thick leathery, pointed at tip; nerves quite prominent. Flowers small, fleshy, pale or dull white, in clusters near the ends of branches, stalks of flowers bent downwards, covered with brownish hair. Flowers strongly musk-scented, falling at dawn. Fruit 2.5-53.5 cm long.

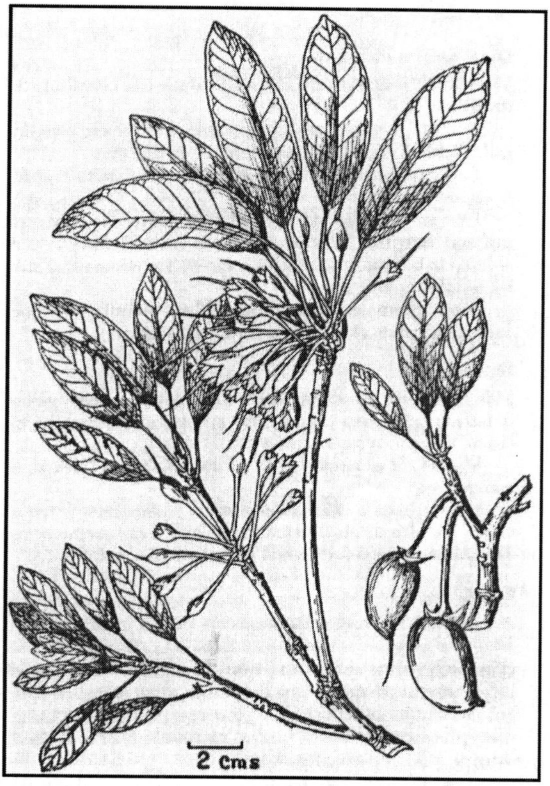

Fig. 19. Madhuca (Madhuca indica).

Distribution : The tree occurs in all the plains and lower hills of India up to 1,200 m; it is very common in submontane regions of the Himalayas, and is at certain places, a chief constitutent of the forest vegetation.

Drug and its Properties : The bark, leaves, flowers and seeds of the tree constitute the drug.

Decoction of the bark is applied in curing itch, bleeding gums and ulcers; it is given internally in diabetes.

Leaves are astringent, their ash, mixed with butter (ghee), is aplied on burns and scalds.

Flowers are used in cough and bronchitis, they are cooling and nutritive. A spirit prepared from flowers is considered to be tonic and nutritive. Flowers possess some antibacterial property.

Seeds promote formation and flow of milk. Oil from seeds is good on skin diseases and as laxative.

Other Uses : Mahua flowers are eaten raw or cooked; their excessive use is harmful. Flowers are largerly employed for making alcohol, vinegar, syrups, jams, etc.

Mahua oil is largely used in manufacture of soaps, in cooking, etc.

Mahua cake is used as manure; sometimes it is fed to cattle. It is also applied to tennis courts to evict earthworms. The timber is used for several miscellaneous purposes.

Other Species : Another very closely allied species of the genus, namely *Madhuca longifolia* (Koening) Macb. syn. *Bassia longifolia* (Koening) occurs in Deccan peninsula and goes under same local name as *M. indica.* The properties of all the plant parts are also similar, and the Indian Pharmaceutical Codex recognises products from both trees as constituents of the official drug.

KAMELA[74]

Mallotus Philippensis (Lamk.) Muell. - Arg.

Family : Euphorbiaceae.

Indian names : Hindi–*Kamela, Rohini, Senduri.*

Description : A small or middle-sized evergreen tree, sometimes only a much-branched large shrub; young parts densely covered with minute red hairs. Leaves alternate, borne on long stalks, variable in shape, 7-20 cm long, their lower side dotted with reddish glands, prominently veined. Flowers minute, male and female on separate plants. Female flowers in erect 5-8 cm long. drooping bunches. Fruit 8-13 mm, roundish, 3-lobed, densely covered with a reddish brown, powdery substance, and minute hair, which are easily rubbed out.

Distribution : The tree is found throughout tropical regions of India from an altitute of 1,500 m in the Himalayas, southwards up to Kerala.

Drug and its Properties : The red glandular and hairy substance separated from the fruits forms the drug.

Kamela is chiefly used for destroying tapeworms. The *Kamela* powder is taken with milk or curd, etc. If one dose of *Kamela* does not expel the worm, the dose is repeatd. Sometimes a dose of castor oil is necessary to expel the dead worm.

Kamela itself is a purgative. It is also used externally in treatment of skin diseases like ringworm and scabies, etc.

The hair on the fruits have been tried (on animals) as oral contraceptives; they have been found to reduce fertility in female rats and guinea-pigs.

Other Uses : The tree is a well-known source of *Kamela* dye and used in colouring textiles.

The oil extracted from seeds is being used in paints and varnishes, and in several other ways. Due to excellent drying properties the oil is much valued in painting work and is in great demand.

The wood of the tree is used for minor domestic articles and fuel; it is suitable for matchboxes. The leaves provided good fodder. The seed cake is used as manure. The bark of the tree contains tannins and is used for tanning leather.

As the local name in certain languages indicates, the red *Kamela* powder is used by women as *Sendur* (Vermillion).

MINT[75]

(*Podina*)

Mentha species.

Family : Lamiaceae.

Indian names : Most of the Indian local names of *Mentha* species are based on the word *Podina*.

The plants belonging to the genus *Mentha* are aromatic herbs. Several species grow wild; some are cultivated. The chif constituents for which these plants are valued are Menthol and Peppermint oil.

Mentha aroensis L. (English–Field Mint, Corn Mint; Indian name–*Podina*) is anerect branched herb upto about 60 cm high. Leaves up to 5 cm long; leafstalk small or none, margins toothed. Flowers small, lilac, in small bunches, borne on axils of leaves.

This herb occurs in Kashmir at an altitude of about 1,500-3,000 m; it is also cultivated.

Infusion of its leaves is used in rheumatic pains and indigestion.

A Japanese variety of this plant (named M. arvensis L. subsp. haplocalyx Briq. var. piperascens Holmes) has been cultivated in Jammu and Kashmir. This yields an oil; its trade name is Japanese Mint Oil or Japanese peppermint Oil. It is used as a substitute for true Peppermint Oil (obtained from M. Piperita).

Mentha longifolia (L.) Huds. (Syn. M. sylvestris L., English–Horsemint, Hindi–*Jangli Podina,* PUnjabi–Koshu) is a larger herb and occurs in Kashmir and northern parts of Punjab and Uttar Pradesh. This plant is considered antiseptic, stimulant, and useful in digestive complaints and fever.

True Peppermint : The most important plant of this group is *Mentha pipcrita* L. (English–Peppermint, Punjabi–*Vilayati Podina*). This plant is cultivated in several parts of India, e.g. in Kashmir, Uttar Pradesh, Mysore, Madras, etc.

The dried leaves and flowering tops of the plant constitute the drug *Peppermint.* The drug is used in treatment of flatulence, vomiting, dirarrhoea and nausea. Bruised leaves are aplied in headache and other pains.

The main use of this drug is for extraction of Peppermint Oil (which contains Menthol) and is largely usd in medicine for stomach disorders, in ointments for headaches, rheumatic and other pains and in cough drops, inhalations, mouth washes, etc. The oil is also antiseptic.

JATAMANSI[76]

(*Spikenard*)

Nardostachys Grandiflora DC. syn. N. jatamansi DC.

Family : Valerianaceae.

Indian names : Hindi–*Jatamansi.*

The trade name is based on the Indian name of the plant. i.e. *Jatamansi,* which refers to the bearded appearance of rhizomes.

Description : A perennial herb up to about 60 cm tall, rhizomes woody, long, covered with fibres from petioles of withered leaves. Lower basal leaves up to about 20 cm long; narrowed into the petiole; upper leaves much smaller, almost ovate. Flowers small, several in small bunches. Fruit small, covered with minute hair.

Distribution : The plant occurs in the alpine Himalayas between 3,000 mand 4,500 m altitude, eastwards to Bhutan.

Drug and its Properties : The dried rhizomes and roots of this plant are medicinal.

Jatamansi has tonic, antispasmodic and stimulant properties; it is therefore, useful in treatment of certain types of fits, convulsions and palpitation of heart. It is used also as laxative and for improving urination, menstruation and digestion.

It is used as a substitute for the drug *Valerian* (*Valeriana officinalis* L.).

Higher altitudes in Himalayas are considered suitable for its cultivation.

TULSI[77]

(*Sacred Basil, Holy Basil*)

ocimum sanctum L.

Family : Lamiaceae.

Indian names : Hindi–*Tulsi.*

Description : This is well-known sacred plant of the Indians. It is a muchbranched erect herb, up to about 75 cm high, hairy all over. Leaves Leaves opposite, about 5 cm long, margins entire or toothed, hairy on upper as well as lower surface, dotted with minute glands, aromatic. Flowers small, purplish or reddish, in small compact clusters on slender spikes. Fruits small, seeds yellowish or reddish.

Description : This plant is grown in houses, gardens, and temples all over India and is often found as escape.

Drug and its Properties : The leaves and seeds of the plant are medicinal.

The oil obtained from leaves has the property of destroying bacteria and insects. The juice or infusion of the leaves is useful in bronchitis, digestive complaints, it is applied locally on ringworm and other skin diseases, it is dropped in ears to relieve earache. A decoction of leaves is used in Indian homes to cure common colds. Seeds are useful in complaints of urinary system. Decoction of root is given in malarial fever to bring about sweating.

Other Uses : The plant is rather an essential article in the worship of Hindu gods and goddesses.

Other Species: ***Ocimum canum*** Sims (English-Hoary Basil, Hindi-*Kali Tulsi, Ram Tulsi, Bharbhari)* is found almost throughout India, generally near habitations, agricultural fields and in waste places. Its seeds are black. Seeds are considered to be tonic and diuretic. The oil from its leaves has similar properties as the oil from O. *sanctum*.

O. *basilicum* L. (English-Sweet Basil, Hindi-*Bubai Tulsi Sabzah*, Sanskrit-Munjariki, Tttamil-Karpura Tulsi) occurs naturally in north-western India andis cultivated in other parts of India. This plant is useful in fever, cough, worms, stomach complaints and gout. Juice of leaves is used as a nasal douche and is applied in skin diseases. Seeds, given internally, relieve constipation and piles.

An exotic East African species of this genus, namely, O. kilmandscharicum Guerke (Camphor Basil) has recently gained much importance as a source of Camphor (Plate III). It has been cultivated in India in Kashmir, Uttar Pradesh, West Bengal, Maharashtra, Mysore, Madras and Kerala. Areas up to an altitude of about 1,000 m are considered suitable for its cultivation. The Terai region of U.P. is very suitable for it. Camphor is largely used in medicine, chiefly in preparations for local application on pains, sprains, etc. (See Cinnamomum camphora).

Camphor is put to several miscellaneous uses. It is mt partly from our own resources and partly from imports.

TURPETH[78]

(Indian Jalap)

OPERCULI NA TURPETHUM (L.) Silva Manso- MERREMIA TURPETHUM (L.) Shahand Bhatt.

Family: Convolvulaceae.

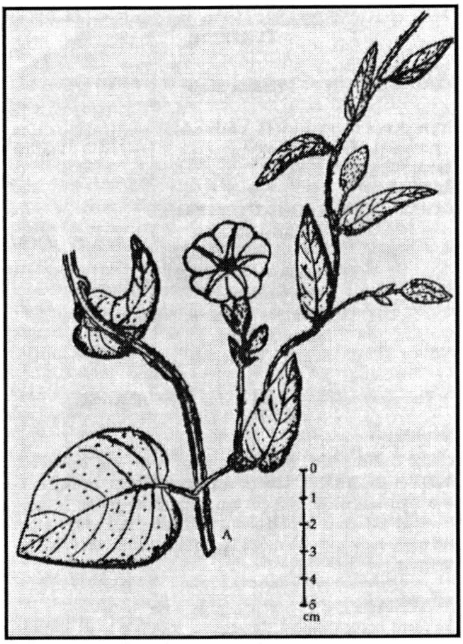

Fig. 20. Turpeth (Operculina Turpethum).

Indian names: Hindi–*Nisoth, Pithori.*

A large twining herb with milky juice, root long, branched, fleshy, stems winged. Leaves 4-10 by 1.5-7 cm, ovate, cor-date. Flowers white, 4-5 cm long, funnel-shaped, in few-flowered bunches. Sepals about 2 cm long, but when plant is in fruit, they become much larger and brittle and enclose the fruits.

Description : The plant occurs almost throughout India up to an altitude of about 1,000 m, it is sometimes grown in gardens for its beautiful flowers.

Drug and its Properties : The dried roots of the plant constitute the drug, the roots should be taken from white variety only, and they should have their bark intact.

The drug contains Turpethin. The *Turpeth* has almost same properties as the true *Jalap,* obtained from *Exogoniumpurga* and is a suitable substitute for it. It is used as a purgative. Powdered roots are suitable for this. The samples of *Turpeth* commonly available in markets have stems and twigs of the plant mixed with the roots.

HARMAL[79]

PEGANUM HARMALA L.

Family : Rutoceae.

Indian names : Hindi–*Gandhya, Harmal.*

Description: A shrub about 30-90 cm high, leaves 5-8 cm long, divided into numerous narrow segments. Flowers 2-3 cm diameter, white, single in axils of leaves. Fruits capsular, globose, 5-8 mm diameter, deeply lobed. Seeds 2.5-4 mm long, brownish, of various shapes and with reticulated seed coat.

Distribution: The plant is found almost throughout northern and northwestern India, and in drier regions of the Deccan.

Drug and its Properties : The dried seeds of the plant constitute the drug *Harmal.*

The seeds contain several alkaloids and are useful in asthma, hysteria, rheumatism, gallstones, colic pains, fever jaundice and complaints of difficult and painful menstruation. They are used also as narcotic, anthelmintic and emetic.

The alkaloids Harmaline, Yageine and Harmine, obtained from this drug, are all psychomimetics, i.enact as hallucinogens. The drug stimulates moter tracts of cerebrum and central nervous system. Higher doses. Are poisonous and bring about severe depressant action on the nervous system.

Experiments have confirmed bactericidal action of the drug, but tests in hospitals did not show any useful effect of the drug in malaria.

Other Uses : The seeds yield a red dye. Powdered roots mixed in mustard oil kill lice in hair. The plant. Kept in a room repels mosquitoes.

PERGULARIA[80]

PERGULARIA DAEMIA (Forsk.) Chiov

Syn. P. *extensa* N. E. Br, *Daemia extensa* R. Br.

Family: Asclepiadaceae.

Indian names : Hindi–*Sadovani, Utarni, Utran.*

Description : A twining herb, stem hairy and with milky juice. Leaves 4-6 cm long, sometimes more. Ovate or round, hairy on lower surface, deeply cordate at base. Flowers pale or white, small, in short clusters. Fruits reflexed in pairs, 5-8 cm long, 1.3 cm broad, covered with spinous outgrowths.

Description : The plant is found almost throughout India up to 1,000 m.

Drug and its Properties *:* The entire plant is used in medicine

The juice of the leaves is given in catarrhal affection and infantile diarrhoea. It forms a constitutent of a purgative preparation given in rheumatism and amenorrhoea. It is used as a uterine tonic, expectorant and emetic. Its action as a uterine tonic has been confirmed experimentally: it is useful is curing gynaecological conditions, such as excessive bleeding, etc. The active principles of pergularia resemble Pituitrin in their action.

PICRORHIZA[81]

(Kutki)

PICRORHIZA KURROOA Royle ex Benth.

Family : Scrophulariaceae.

Indian names : Hindi-*Kuru, Kutki.*

Description : It is a small herb with spathula-shaped, 5-10 cm long leaves. Rhizomes of the plant are 15-25 cm long and woody. Flowers small, in cylindric spikes, spikes borne on almost leafless erect stems. Flowers are of two kinds, some are with 8 mm long filaments. Fruits 1.3 cm long.

Distribution: The plant occurs only in highly mountains, i. E. at about 3,000-4,000 m altitude in the Himalayas from Kashmir to Sikkim.

Drugs and its Properties : The drug comprises the dried rhizomes of the plant.

It is bitter tonic and is useful as antiperiodic and promotes secretion of bile. It is believed to have same properties as *Gentian,* i. E. improves appetite and stimulates gastric secretion. It is also used in dropsy.

The antibiotic activity of the drug *picrorhiza* has been shown experimentally.

The Himalayan mountains between the altitudes of 3,000 and 4,000 m are considered to

PINE[82]

(*Chil*)

PINUS ROXBURGHII Sargent syn. P. *longifolia* Roxb.

Family : Coniferae

Indian names : Hindi—*Chir-Chil.*

The specific name *roxburghii* is in honour of the wellknown botanist Roxburgh, who is called 'Father of Indian Botany'.

Description : It is a large tree with typical needle leaves, leaves 25-30 cm long, in clusters of three, Male cones small, female fruiting cones 10-20 cm long, conical.

Drugs and its Properties : The drug *Oil of Turpentine* is obtained by purification form turpentine, an oleoresin obtained from P. *roxburghii* and certain other species of this genus.

The oil has local irritant action and most of its medicinal uses are dur to that property. In controlled small doses it acts as a stimulant expectorant colic. It has limited use also in typhoid, minor haemorrhages (such as from gums, nose, etc.) Given as an enema, is as a liniment in rheumatic pains. Inhaling the vapours of turpentine is useful in bronchitis.

Other Uses : The timber of the tree is largely used for various purposes, e.g. house-building, furniture, tea chests, match industry, sports goods, musical instruments, etc.

Its resin *Biroja* is used for bangles. The bark has tannins and colouring matter.

LONG PEPPER[83]

PIPER LONGUM L.

Family: Piperaceae.

Indian names : Hindi—*Pipal, Pipali.*

The trade name *Long Pepper* is based on the common English name Pepper. It is called *Long Pepper* as its spikes are long and distinguish it from the other important species of the genus, P. *nigrum* L. whose fruits are round.

In some early literature *Long Pepper* is referred to by the name 'Magadhi' which denotes that the plant is indigenous to the region of Magadh (i.e. Noeth Bihar).

Description : A small aromatic plant trailing on ground, also climbing. Lower leaves 6-10 cm long, broadly ovate, deeply cordate with big lobes at base, upper leaves oblong-ovate, cordate, all dark green and shining above, pale on lower surface, stipules conspicuous, 1.3. cm long, but soon falling. Spikes of flowers solitary, bracts of male spikes narrow, of female circular. Fruit small ovoid, sunk in fleshy spike which is 2.5-4 cm, ovoid, oblong, blackish green, shining.

Distribution: The plant grows in warmer regions of India and is also cultivated.

Drug and its Properties : Long Pepper consists of the dried fruits of the plant.

It is used as a tonic, and in making irritating snuffs. It is also used in Iniments for rheumatic pains and paralysis. A decoction made from the dried immature fruits is useful in chronic bronchitis. Ripe fruits are aromatic, stomachic and carminative.

The antibiotic activity of the leaves and fruits has been shown experimentally.

Other Uses : Another very important species of the genus is *Piper nigrum* L. or *Black Pepper* (Bengali, Hindi—*Gol Mirch, Kali Mirch, Dakhnimirch*, Sanskrit—*Kaphvirodhi* Madras—*Kalluvalh)* Most of the vernacular names of the plant describe the shape (Gol—round) or colour (Kali—black) of the fruits. The Sanskrit name indicates the use of the plant.

P. *nigrum* is a robust woody climber with large, broad, ovate or round leaves. Flowers borne in long spikes, fruits small, globose, 6-7 mm diameter, yellow, turning red when ripe.

The dried unripe fruits constitute the drug *Black Pepper*. It is stimulant, carminative and stomachic, taken in larger quantities, it gives a feeling of warmth and causes sweating. It is also diuretic but can cause irritation in urinary tract. Certain experiments on seeds have shown antibiotic activity of seeds.

The *Black Pepper* is used in may culinary preparations as a condiment and carminative.

Piper cubeba L.f. *(Cubeb, Shitalchini, Sugandhmaricha, Kababchini)* is a native of South-east Asia, its fruits yield an oil which is useful in complaints of urinary system. Eastern and southern India are considered suitable for its cultivation.

ISHABGUL[84]

Plate IV

PLANTAGO OVATA Forsk.

Family: Plantaginaceae

Indian names: The local cames of this plant in different regions and languages of India are only minor variations of the Sanskrit word *Ishapgola or Ishabgul.*

The trade name is also based on that word.

Description : An almost stemless small herb, covered with dense or soft hairy growth. Leaves 8-25 cm long, very narrow. Flowers minute, in oval or cylindric spikes, 1.5-4 cm long. 8 mm long, its upper half separates like a lid. Seeds boat-shaped.

Distribution : The plant grows naturally in only restricted areas in north western India, but is largely cultivated elsewhere.

Drug and its Properties : The seeds of this plant (as also of certain other species of the genus) constitute the drug.

The useful properties of the seeds are due chiefly to the large amount of mucilage and albuminous matter present in them.

Ishabgul is very useful in several kinds of chronic dysentery, such as of amoebic and bacillary origin and chronic diarrhoeas. It is useful as a soothing agent for mucous membranes, and is useful in constipation. Seeds should be soaked in water before use, so that they soon get disintegrated in the alimentary canal, else the whole seeds can cause irritation or even mechanical obstruction in intestines. The large amount of mucilage in the seeds, 'binds' and increases the mass of the stool, and smoothens its passing out. The action is however, chiefly mechanical, rather than physiological.

Ishabgul husk (Hindi—*Ishabgul-ki-bhusi*) is the dry seedcoat of *Plantago ovata,* obtained by crushing the seeds and separating the husk by winnowing.

The husk has the same properties as seeds, rather it has the advantage that there is no risk of mechanical obstruction or irritation in alimentary canal by the husk. The husk, therefore, is taken without any presoaking and is more easy to use than the whole seeds.

The embryo oil of seeds having 50 per cent linoleic acid prevents arteriosclerosis. Oil is more active than safflower oil, and was found to reduce the serum cholesterol level in rabbits.

References

1. Workshop on Medicinl Plants to focus Small farmers- Ch. Prashant Reddy- Hyderabad, June 5. The Business Line, June 6, 2000. p. 1 (The National Institute of Rural Development Hyderabad conducted 2 days workshop on the topic disseminating technical, managerial and financial information on Medicinal and Aromatic Plants so as to facilited small and marginal farmers to take up cultivation on the crops.
2. *Ibid.,* p. 2.
3. *Ibid.,* p. 2.
4. *Ibid.,* p. 2.
5. *Ibid.,* p. 2.
6. *Ibid.,* p. 2.
7. A. Subhbiah, A. Malaisamy and C. Ravindra, India Herbal Industry-Issues and Challenges pp. 1-4 at 4-1-2004.
8. Narain Singh Chauhan, Medicinal and Aromtic Plants of Himachal Pradesh, India Publicshing Company, 1999 p. 47.
9. *Ibid.,* p. 49.
10. *Ibid.,* p. 52.
11. *Ibid.,* p. 56.
12. *Ibid.,* p. 59.
13. *Ibid.,* p. 62.
14. *Ibid.,* p. 56.
15. *Ibid.,* p. 59.
16. *Ibid.,* p. 62.
17. *Ibid.,* p. 65.
18. *Ibid.,* p. 69.
19. *Ibid.,* p. 72.

20. *Ibid.,* p. 76.
21. *Ibid.,* p. 80.
22. *Ibid.,* p. 83.
23. *Ibid.,* p. 90.
24. *Ibid.,* p. 91.
25. *Ibid.,* p. 94.
26. *Ibid.,* p. 96.
27. Medicinal plant S. K. Jain, National Book Trust India A- 5, Green Park, New Delhi - 16, 2001 Saka 1922, p. 18.
28. *Ibid.,* p. 11.
29. *Ibid.,* p. 20.
30. *Ibid.,* p. 07.
31. *Ibid.,* p. 27.
32. *Ibid.,* p. 29.
33. *Ibid.,* p. 31.
34. *Ibid.,* p. 34.
35. *Ibid.,* p. 36.
36. *Ibid.,* p. 40.
37. *Ibid.,* p. 42.
38. *Ibid.,* p. 44.
39. *Ibid.,* p. 47.
40. *Ibid.,* p. 47.
41. *Ibid.,* p. 49.
42. *Ibid.,* p. 51.
43. *Ibid.,* p. 53.
44. *Ibid.,* p. 54.
45. *Ibid.,* p. 56.
46. *Ibid.,* p. 62.
47. *Ibid.,* p. 61.
48. *Ibid.,* p. 62.
49. *Ibid.,* p. 63.
50. *Ibid.,* p. 65.
51. *Ibid.,* p. 66.
52. *Ibid.,* p. 68.
53. *Ibid.,* p. 70.
54. *Ibid.,* p. 72.

55. *Ibid.*, p. 75.
56. *Ibid.*, p. 77.
57. *Ibid.*, p. 80.
58. *Ibid.*, p. 82.
59. *Ibid.*, p. 88.
60. *Ibid.*, p. 90.
61. *Ibid.*, p. 92.
62. *Ibid.*, p. 94.
63. *Ibid.*, p. 96.
64. *Ibid.*, p. 98.
65. *Ibid.*, p. 100.
66. *Ibid.*, p. 102.
67. *Ibid.*, p. 104.
68. *Ibid.*, p. 106.
69. *Ibid.*, p. 112.
70. *Ibid.*, p. 114.
71. *Ibid.*, p. 116.
72. *Ibid.*, p. 119.
73. *Ibid.*, p. 121.
74. *Ibid.*, p. 123.
75. *Ibid.*, p. 125.
76. *Ibid.*, p. 127.
77. *Ibid.*, p. 130.
78. *Ibid.*, p. 132.
79. *Ibid.*, p. 134.
80. *Ibid.*, p. 136.
81. *Ibid.*, p. 138.
82. *Ibid.*, p. 140.
83. *Ibid.*, p. 194.
84. *Ibid.*, p. 168.

3

Market Potential of Medicinal Plants

(A) MARKET POTENTIAL OF MEDICINAL PLANTS IN INDIA

India represents one of the eight important centres of origin and crop plant diversity of cultivated plants and their wild relatives. It is immensely rich in medicinal and aromatic plants occurring in diverse ecosystems. World Health Organisation (WHO) has listed over 21,000 plant species used around the world for medicinal purposes (National Bureau of Plan Genetic Resources (NBPGR) booklet, 1996).[1] It has been estimated that India has 47,000 species of plants and is No. 8 in world biodiversity. Out of there, medicinal plants comprise of 8,000 species. Indian System of Medicine (ISM) uses around 2,500 plant species belonging to more than 1,000 genera. About 800 species are used by industry of which approximately 25% are cultivated. Exports of herbal materials and medicines can jump from just Rs. 446 crore now to Rs. 3,000 crore by 2005. And, with a "grand strategic plan", exports can shoot to Rs. 10,000 crore by 2010.[2] The international market for such plants is more than $60 billion a year, and growing at a rate of seven per cent.[3] Within the country, these could well provide affordable healthcare and conserve biodiversity. A survey has shown India has more than 8,000 species of medicinal plants, the main healthcare resource for the majority.[4] But unlike China, it just hasn't been able to seize the business opportunity. Just about everything is missing from India's effort: standardisation, quality control and efficacy of drugs, organised marketing and integrated development – from production to consumption – to boost exports. The task force strongly recommends filling the policy vacuum with a medicinal plants board, fuelled by Rs. 50 crore over three years, for integrated development. The sector itself will need

Rs. 1,000 crore over five years. And, the possibility of external funding may be explored to ensure health for all' by 2005. While doing all this, India will need to move fast to protect its traditional knowledge the priority has to be a digital database of such knowledge. And, modernisation of patent efforts. Task force members say India already has the expertise: Medicinal plants are used in homes, there are 1.5 million practitioners of traditional medicine systems, about 4.6 lakh registered practitioners and more than 8,000 registered pharmacies of Indian systems of medicine and homeopathy.[5] Nine – tenths of the plants are collected from the wild, generating about 40 million madness of employment.[6] The flip side: Since nearly three-fourths of collection involves destructive harvesting, many plants are endangered. They are collected without paying attention to their maturity and stored haphazardly for long periods under unsuitable conditions which ensure rejection by importers and standard manufacturing drug units. Since the gatherers generally get a low price, they often "mine" the plants – ultimately, at some cost to themselves. For, as forest habitats disappear and stocks of wild medicinal plant material go down, there's "a corresponding drop in the availability of plants used as the first and last resort for all healthcare by the rural population". Pharmacies are owned mostly by family companies. Marketing is "inefficient, informal, secretive and opportunistic. As a result, the raw material supply situation is shaky, unsustainable and exploitative. This results in depletion of resource base, exploitation of rural people (who are the real stewards of the resource), adulteration and non-availability of quality herbal drugs for domestic consumption as well as exports."

Despite convincing progress in Synthetic Chemistry and Biotechnology, plants are the most important sources for preventive and curative medical preparations. WHO has estimated that at least 80% of all the global inhabitants rely on curative medical systems of medicine for there are four well-recognised systems of traditional medicine namely, Ayurveda, Unani, Siddha and Yoga and Naturopathy.[7]

Medicinal plant species are, still to large extent, gathered and collected from the wild and relatively few genera are cultivated on a commercial scale. This exploitation coupled with increasing urbanisation led to a steady erosion and loss of diversity from the natural habitats of these plants. Thus rapid loss of natural forests is more worrisome in regard to loss of plants with as yet undiscovered pharmaceuticals. Upto 1990, 47 major drugs have been developed from the tropical plants.[8]

Overall, 119 plants derived prescription drugs are commonly used in different countries, 74 per cent of which were discovered due to chemical isolation of active compounds of plants used in traditional systems of medicines.[9] Examples include cardiac glycosides Digoxin and derivatives from Digitalis purpure, used in European traditional medicines, Reserpine, a tranquilise r and anti-hypertensive agent from Rauwolfia serpentine known for its value in Ayurveda.[10]

Since majority of the medicinal plants are collected from the wild by the unskilled people, problems of inconsistent quality, adulteration, destructive method of collection leading to extinction or endangered status of number of plants, are severe. On the other hand, the demand for herbal medicines is increasing day by day as more and more people become aware of the dangers of side effects of Allopathic medicines. In order to bridge the gap between these two scenarios, it is necessary to undertake a detailed study to shortlist a few medicinal plants for extensive cultivation and then to concentrate on standardising the cultivation practices, post-harvest technologies related to these plant by adhering to good Agricultural Practices (GAP) and Good Manufacturing Practices (GAP).

Another need of the hour is to develop "value-added production of Herbal and for Phytochemicals" at the community level so that most of the price benefit is achieved at the farmer level rather than the middleman level.

Global trends in production and utilisation

More than 50 commercially important medicinal plants are traded extensively in the international market. Their prices are governed by price levels in markets at Hamburg, New York and Osaka.[11]

Indian Exports to Different Countries

The export of medicinal plants from India is in from forms:

- As dried plants or plant parts. e.g. liquorice roots, Senna leaves, Vinca Rosa (Catharanthus roseus) herbs.
- As extracts e.g. Sag of opium poppy.
- As isolated and purified active ingredients/intermediates e.g. Gymnema powder, Atropise sulphate, menthal crystals, Calcium sennoside.
- As formulations e.g. Over the counter (OTC) drugs, proprietary formulations etc. The total volume of exports

has increased quite substantially from Rs. 612 crores in 1996-1997 to Rs. 6773 crores in 1998-1999.[12] The major contribution to this rise, which is more than ten fold, comes from "Menthol Crystals", the export of which increased from Rs. 74 crores Rs. 3003 crores during this period.[13] The export of Ayurvedic and Unani medicines varied between Rs. 56 crores and Rs. 96 crores.[14] Among herbs and plants, Ginseng roots, Isabgul husk and Senna leaves and pods dominate. USA, Federal Republic of Germany, UK, France, Switzerland, Japan, Italy and Netherlands account for majority of the Indian exports followed by Asian and African countries. It is also clear that India is exporting very less number of "Value-Added Products" and the main focus is on the export of dried plants or plants or powders.

Marketing Channel

Medicinal Plants are mostly collected in wild. They are purchased by traders and then sold again either to exporters or to industry. The export of medicinal plants is also in raw from either by way of roots, branches, barks, etc, or crude extraction powders.

Vision for the Future Global Trends and Perspectives

As stated earlier, the early part of the 20th century brought an evaluation of pharmaceutical industry. With the progress in chemical techniques, crude drugs came to be replaced in the pharmaceutical industry by pure chemical drugs and the developed countries witnessed a decline in popularity of medicinal plant therapy. But the present developments indicate that, in these countries, the pendulum has swung again and there is a resurgence of interest in study and use of medicinal plants. They are increasingly used as (1) source of direct therapeutic agents, (2) as a raw material based for the elaboration of more complex semi-synthetic chemical compounds, (3) as models for new synthetic compounds and (4) as taxonomic markets for the discovery of new compounds.

The production, consumption and international trade in medicinal plants, and phytomedicines are, therefore, expected to grow at more than the historical rate of 7 per cent per year.

Opportunities present themselves in two ways

Increasing market size, both national and global, for plant based products: As described earlier, this market is increasing due to limitations of modern medicine, new discoveries/ rediscoveries of several medicinal properties of plants and herbs, and larger reach of health services to people. The rise in cosmetic and health food industry is also contributing to this increase. India can and must take a larger share of this market.

Increasing research capability: With its wealth of knowledge on medicinal plants and herbs India is the most suitable candidate for fundamental and application-oriented research in this field. In fact, next to Information Technology and Biotechnology, research in medicinal plants, which combines both these technologies, should emerge as the most sustainable growth sector in the years to come.

Short Listing of Plants in India

For the purpose of short listing following selection criteria have been adopted:

The endemic nature of plants, high domestic as well as export demand, Endangered nature of the plant, Documented use in traditional systems of medicines.

Aloe vera (Ghrita Kumari): It acts as a source of nourishment for HIV patients, stimulates immune response against cancer. The gel and powder from Aloe vera has great international demand.

Bacopa mannieri (Brahmi): This is an aquatic plants community found in rice fields. Numerous scientific studies conducted by Central Drug Institute of India (CDRI) have shown Bacopa to improve learning ability, retention and enhance results. Results of these studies were presented to world community at the International Brain Research Conferences during 1986-1996. It showed the following activities:

- Faster Performance times, reduction in errors, improved acquisition and retention of learning, decreased forgetfulness, increased ability to adapt to new learning.

Centella asiatica (Mandookparni, Goty kola): It has the ability to rebuild energy reserves. For this region, it is called 'food for the brain'. It increases mental and physical power. It combats stress and improves reflexes.

Rauwolfia serpentina (Sarpagandha): Sarpagandha is a tropical evergreen climbing shrub. It was used for centuries to treat insanity as well as physical illnesses such as fevers and snakebites. The thick dry roots yield alkaloids like Reserpine.

Cantharanthus roseus: This is a small plant yielding a number of clinically alkaloids. Out of these Vincristine and Vinblastine are used to treat leukemia. They have a large global demand.

Taxus baccata/T. wallichiana (Himalayan yew): This is a slow growing tree from the Himalayas, found in restricted locations above a height of 2000 m.

Impact of International Trade

There is large-scale international trade in medicinal plants, used both for herbal medicine and for the manufacture of pharmaceutical drugs. There is also growing interest in obtaining samples of plant material, or traditional knowledge about plants uses, to explore for new commercial medical products. The scale of international trade in medicinal plants is difficult to assess, because of a paucity of reliable statistics and trade secrecy, but it is growing rapidly.

India ranks second after China developing countries in export of pharmaceuticals and is ahead of such technologically advanced countries as Mexico, South Korea, Brazil, Israel etc.

Improved technological capability is also reflected in terms of the ability of India to raise her share in patents granted by the US patents office from 0.02 per cent in 1977-87 period to 0.06 per cent during 1996-2000. Although still having marginal sharing in the US patent grants, India has not faced badly compared to other developing countries. In 1998, it ranked seventh amongst all developing countries in terms of the magnitude of US patents obtained, behind Taiwan, South Korea and Israel- the three leading nations but ahead of Brazil, China and Mexico. Interestingly, in the chemical sector which accounts for the bulk of all patents- and in biotechnology-one of the cutting edge sectors-India ranks fourth amongst developing countries. Moreover, in biotechnology, the gap between India and countries ahead of it is not large.

The increasing technological capability is terms of rising exports of drugs and pharmaceuticals. With their cost effective process innovations, Indian companies have emerged as competitive suppliers in the world of a large number of generic drugs that are now outside the patent protection.

That has resulted in a steady growth of India's exports of drugs and pharmaceuticals. Thus the industry has evolved has evolved from one being highly import dependent to one that generates increasing export surplus for the country. The faster growth of pharmaceutical exports has resulted in their share in India's exports rising from 0.55 per cent in 1970-71 to over 4 per cent by the 1999-2000.

Emerging comparative advantage of India in pharmaceuticals is apparent from Table 1 which shows that India's share in world exports of pharmaceuticals has risen by 2.5 times while her share in all merchandise exports has stagnated at about 0.6 per cent throughout the 1970 to 1998 period.

Table 3.1. India's Pharmaceutical Exports in World Trade, 1970 to 1998 (Current prices) (in Rs. crore)

Year	*Share of India in World Exports*	
	All Merchandise	*Pharmaceuticals*
1970	0.6	0.4
1975	0.5	0.4
1980	0.4	0.8
1985	0.5	0.8
1990	0.5	1.2
1995	0.6	1.0
1997	0.6	1.1
1998	0.6	1.0

Indian exports of pharmaceuticals received a boost in the late 1980s when a number of drugs went off the patents and Indian companies manufacturing them with cost-effective processes entered the international markets after obtaining FDA approval. Therefore, in the late 1980s, as much as 61 per cent of India's pharmaceutical exports bulk drugs.

However, subsequently some of larger and more dynamic India enterprises such as Ranbaxy Laboratories, Dr. Reddy's Labs, Cipla and Cadila, have started marketing their own formulations in different countries with the help of a growing network of overseas offices and subsidiaries set up in key international markets. As a result, the share of bulk drugs in total exports of pharmaceuticals has come down to around 40 per cent.

In analysis, we have relied on price (Rs. per kg.) currently prevailing in different markets of the country, to enlist the top twenty medicinal plants. This list (Table 2) has been complied after a thorough review of plants drugs or botanicals, across the major raw drugs or botanicals, across the major raw drug markets of India, selling at prices of at least Rs. 100/kg. of dry material. The plant sources of these top twenty raw drugs have been identified and enlisted.

Table 3.2. Highly demanded top 20 Medicinal Plants Traded in India

Sl. No.	*Trade Name*	*Botanical Name*	*Part used*
1.	Atis	Aconitum heterophllum Wall. Ex Royle	Tuberous roots
2.	Meetha telia/ Bachnag	Aconitum violoceum (Jacq.) Stapf	Tuberous roots
3.	Safed Musali	Chiorophytum borivllianum Sant. and Fernandez	Tubers
4.	Guggul	Commiphora wightii (A) Bhandari	Resin
5.	Nanura/Mishmi-Bitter	Coptis teeta Wall.	Roots
6.	salam panja/salep	Dactylorhiza hatagirea (D. Don.) Soo	Tubers
7.	vidanga/baibaranga	Embelia ribes Burm. f.	Fruits
8.	Nagkesar	Mesua nagassarium (Burm. F.) Kostern	Dry Stamens
9.	Rampatri/Bombay Mace	Myristica malabarica Lam.	Aril and Mace
10.	Jatamansi	Nardostachys grandiflora DC.	Rhizomes and roots
11.	Gaozagan	Onosma Bractearum Wall.	Flowers
12.	Kutki	Picrorhiza kurrooa Royle ex Benth	Roots and Rhizomes
13.	Kakra-Singi	Pistacia integerrima Stewart ex brandis	Galls
14.	Sarpagandha	Rauvolfia serpentina Benth. ex Kurz	Roots
15.	Manjishta	Rubia cordifolia Linn.	Roots
16.	Chandana/Sandalwood	Santalum album Linn.	Heartwood
17.	Chobchini Gulabi	Smilax glabra Roxb.	1 Roots
18.	Chiraiyita	Swertia chirayita Karst.	Whole Plant
19.	Taggar/Mushkbala	Valeriana hardwickii Wall.	Rhizomes and Roots
20.	Banafsha	Viola pilosa Blume	Flowers

The Table 3 shows the important medicinal plants, which are imported from aboard. The reason for importing this medicinal plants may be lack of availability of these plants in India or not much awareness of their technology in India.

Table 3.3. Medicinal Plants being Imported

Botanical Name	*Canway Name*
Glycyrrhiza glabra	Mullathi
Pimpinella aniswn	Anise fruit
Thymus vulgaris	Hasha
Operculina turpenthum	Turbud
Cuscuta epithymum	Aftimurn vilaiyti
Smilax omata	Ushba
S. China	Chobchini
Lavandula stoechas	Ustukhudus

Table shows major industries in medicinal plants trade in our country. There are 25 companies involved in medicinal plants trade in India.

Table 3.4. India Pharma Companies Diversified / Marketing Herbal Products

Sl. No	*Companies*
1.	Albert David Ltd.
2.	Alembic Chemical Works Co. Ltd.
3.	Biological E. Ltd.
4.	Cadila Healthcare Pvt. Ltd.
5.	Cadila Pharmaceuticals Ltd.
6.	Cipla Ltd.
7.	Concept Pharmaceuticals Ltd.
8.	Croslands
9.	Deepharma Ltd.
10.	Dey's Medical Stores (Mfg.) Ltd.
11.	Dr. Reddy's Lab.
12.	East India Pharmaceuticals Ltd.

Sl. No	*Companies*
13.	Elders Pharma
14.	Franco-Indian Pharmaceuticals Ltd.
15.	Gufic Ltd.
16.	J.B. Chemicals Pharmaceutical Ltd.
17.	Lupin laboratories Ltd.
18.	Lyka Labs. Ltd.
19.	Merind Ltd.
20.	Parke-Davis (India) Ltd.
21.	Rallis India Ltd.
22.	Ranbaxy Laboratories Ltd.
23.	Themis (Phytomedica)
24.	TTK Parma Pvt. Ltd.
25.	Wockhardt Ltd.

Conclusion

Conservation issues in international trade in medicinal plants for existing products mainly concern those plants which are harvested from the 'wild' which is the case for the great majority of species.

Conservation issues arise if the trade threatens conservation of biodiversity or is not sustainable. Biodiversity or is not sustainable. Biodiversity may be threatened if the trade endangers survival of the species, erodes its genetic diversity or cause loss or degradation of important natural or semi-natural ecosystems.

The international movement of plant samples (or traditional knowledge about the uses of plants) for analysis to discover possible new commercial products raises the issue of equitable distribution of reward in the event of successful commercialisation. Following the Biodiversity Treaty, there is an urgent need for equitable partnership to be developed between those involved in developing new commercial products from plants and those responsible for conservation of biodiversity (often in the South).

For example, if plants are being over-harvested from wild populations, then potential solutions include the design and implementation of new methods of managing wild populations, or transferring the business to reliance on cultivated plants.

Many botanic gardens, having skills in plant propagation and horticulture, are in a special position to assist with the process of introducing plants into cultivation, but they will generally need to work closely with other agencies better equipped to deal with other necessary aspects, including social and economic ones. Success in making harvesting of species sustainable must involve the social dimension.

Challenges Ahead

- Development of proper inventory and data base bank for medicinal plants of India.
- Detailed chemical investigation of selected plants giving important new leads on novel active molecules.
- Studies on new medicinal plants that can serve as substitutes for other plants with high demand and also for threatened plants.
- Development of in vitro propagation methods for a number of hitherto unstudied plants.
- Development of an effective network of dissemination of information, training and technology transfer and post harvest transfer.
- Development of technology parks and demonstration farms.
- Development of industries near farming areas to give impetus to production of value added product and reduce the stronghold of middleman.
- Development of consortium for collection of raw materials, processing, marketing and export.
- Standardisation of quality parameters for medicinal plants both for domestic and export markets.
- Protection of Intellectual Properly Rights (IPR) at the global scale.

Policy Option

The Government of India and the State Governments have taken many steps to improve the conditions. There re several institutions for conducting research in various aspects of the cultivations and use of medicinal plant. The department of forests have been given instructions to preserve and promote plantation of medicinal herbs. Recently, the Government of India has national set up a 'Medicinal Plants Board' with a corpus of Rs. 100 crores, to promote and regulate supply and export of medicinal herbs in the area of establishing linkages, market development and infrastructure development.

Finances

NABARD should prepare financial guidelines for production, processing and manufacturing for each of selected products and disseminate the information among bankers, farmers, and entrepreneurs. NABARD could even be a nodal agency for arranging a network of producers and manufacturers.

Taxation and Incentives

All taxes, including octroi, excise and sales tax, on the medicinal plants and their products should be abolishes or substantially reduced. No market fees should be collected by the regulated markets on the sale of medicinal herbs through them; instead, twice this amount should be given to them as grant by the State Governments to encourage them to regulate these Commodities. NHB National Horticulture Board and APEDA should extend all their schemes of assistance to the selected medicinal plants.

EXPORT OF MEDICINAL PLANTS IN INDIA

According to the World Health Organisation estimates, the present demand for medicinal plants is about US $14 billion a year and projected dem and by the year 2050 is US$5 trillion. Medicinal plant related trade in India is estimated to be around Rs. 550 crores per year. While the value of global trade in medicinal plants has been put at over $60 billion per year, Indians total turnover of Rs. 2300 crores of Ayurvedic and herbal products, major over-the-counter (OTC) products contribute around Rs. 1200 crores.

Other formulations fetch around Rs. 650 crores. And classical Ayurvedic formulations contribute the remaining Rs. 450 crores. With world demand growing at 1% annually, the export market for medicinal plants appears to be growing faster than the Indian domestic market.

An earlier Exim bank study, finds renewed world wide interest in natural medicines and newer cases in food and cosmetic industries, with good prospects for exports of medicinal plants from India. A favourable policy framework is required to promote commercial cultivation, research and development, and increased exports of medicinal plants. The study adds that exports of finished products, rather than of crude material, should be encouraged.

The cosmetics industry as well as aromatherapy are two

important areas where Indian medicinal plants or their value-added extracts or essential oils can contribute a lot globally. Indian will have to hone its marketing skills with suitable strategies capable of catering to the dynamic market requirements, supported by an appropriate policy framework.

The study also advocates an integrated approach to promote export of medicinal plants from India, right from the stage of research, cultivation, collection, storage, processing and marketing in an organised manner, with the help of leading Indian pharmaceutical companies. It adds that it is imperative to evolve a national policy in medicinal plant conservation, a nationwide network of medicinal plant nurseries.

For long-term conservation and management of medicinal plants, an in situ network would have to be integrated with regular forestry and wild life management in the country. Illustrated manuals and comprehensive lists correlating local and trade names, with botanical names need to be prepared to help international and national efforts to manage trade in wild medicinal plants.

The study advocates strict legislative measures to check indiscriminate exploitation of forest resources, to save many medicinal plant species from extinction.

It finds India in an advantageous position for cultivation, on account of many types of climatic and soil conditions. To maintain standards of quality, safety and move for harmonisation and standardisation with Scientific Data, other measures include the training of pharmacologists in medicinal plants research.

According to a UNIDO study, the following constraints are associated with the use of traditional medicine sector in developing countries including India.

- Poor agricultural practice.
- Poor harvesting and post harvest practice.
- Lack of research on development of high yielding varieties.
- Poor propagation methods.
- Inefficient processing techniques leading to low yields and poor quality products.
- Poor quality control procedures.
- High energy losses during processing.
- Lack of current good manufacturing practices.
- Difficulties in marketing.

- Lack of local market for primary processed products.
- Lack of trained personnel and equipment.
- Lack of facilities to fabricate equipment locally.
- Lack of access to latest technological and market information.

India is sitting on a gold mine of well recorded and well practiced knowledge of traditional herbal medicine. But unlike China, India has not been able to capitalise on this herbal wealth by promoting its use in the developed world despite their renewed interest in herbal medicines. This can be achieved by judicious product identification based on diseases found in the developed world for which no medicine or only palliative therapy is available, such herbal medicines will find speedy access into those countries.

The basic requirements for gaining entry into developed countries include :

1. Well documented traditional use.
2. Single plant medicines.
3. Medicinal plants-free from pesticides, heavy metals etc.
4. Standardisation based on chemical activity profiles, and
5. Safety and stability.

However, mode of action studies in animals and efficacy in human beings will do in order to establish the curative properties of these drugs. Such scientifically generated data will project herbal medicine in a proper perspective and help in getting a sustained global market for the same.

Resource Base

The number of plants that are used medicinally is very large. The Natural Products Alert (NAPRA-LERT) database at the University of Illinois has documented the ethno medicinal uses for more than 9,000 species, including monocotyledons, dicotyledons, gymnosperms, pterid-ophytes, bryophytes and lichens (Farnsworth and Soejarto, 1991).

Uncontrolled Exploitation

Despite all their importance, medicinal plants are, for the moment at least, seldom handled within an organised, regulated sector: most are still exploited with little or no regard to the future. As noted, escalating consumer demand is already resulting in the indiscriminate harvest of wild plants. This is damaging both ecosystems and their precious biodiversity. The damage is especially serious when bark, roots, seeds and flowers all essential for the species survival are removed.

Table 3.5. Natural Medicines Market Regional Growth Rated 1991 – 98 (in percentage)

Region	*1991 – 92*	*1993 – 98*
EU	5	8
Rest of Europe	8	12
SE Asia	12	12
Japan	15	15
South Asia	15	15

It seems unlikely that medicinal plants will decrease in importance anytime soon. For one thing, the number or people demanding greater access to herbal remedies in the industrialised countries seems likely to go increasing. For another, the healing plants will continue as the primary means of preventive and curative healthcare in the developing countries, Indeed, rising population growth and falling economic levels will probably make these plants more important than today.

The present time, therefore, offers a unique opportunity to work with developing countries in implementing policies to regulate medicinal plant conservation, cultivation, processing, and marketing. At this pioneering stage, in which norms and standards for the healthcare of billions of people in the developing nations are going to be rapidly set, a strategy for the future should be developed. This will be far from easy; the medicinal-plant business is fluid, undocumented, and largely unregulated. Much about it is unclear, and will remain that way for some time. But, regardless of the difficulties, a beginning must be made to address this important but neglected area.

A preliminary review of available data on markets and prices- indicates that at present no complete data for even single – medicinal species is available; almost no data on actual production, employment, and pricing, and financial flows between countries is available.

The market prices for medicinal plants and materials derived from them provide only limited insight into the – workings of the markets and their profits. All of these uncertainties need to be taken into account in developing strategies and policies for future decision – making purposes. For many countries, medicinal plants are a possible "bridge" between sustainable economic development, affordable healthcare and the conservation of vital biodiversity.

Acceptance

There is a need to create a greater awareness of the medicinal and economic value of medicinal plants within and outside the country. This is especially important among government officials, farmers, and scientists.

Tradition is especially important in the case of medicinal plants. Any strategy to preserve such species will have to take people's needs and perceptions into account. Local users often have a good understanding of how sustainable harvesting should be practiced (Cunningham, 1991).

In China, plant – based medicine id the backbone of the health care for perhaps a billion people; botanicals are used for the primary health care need of 40 per cent of China's urban patients and over 90 per cent of its rural patients.

Institutional Capacities

At present few developing countries have the resources or institutional capability to advise on policy and regulatory mechanisms and to provide the level of research required to guarantee a production of medicinal plants to sustain local pharmaceutical industries and provide for healthcare needs. The subject tends to fall into two government ministries that normally don't deal directly with each other: agriculture and health. They would have to coordinate programmes if medicinal plants are to be cultivated.

Table 3.6. Distribution of Medicinal Plants by Habit (based on analysis of 1079 South Indian species)

Habit	*Number*	*Percentage*
Herbs	344	32
Shrubs	220	20
Trees	354	33
Climbers	127	12
Others	34	3

Source : FRLHT.

Table 3.7. Distribution of Medicinal Plants by Parts used (based on analysis of 1079 South Indian species)

Parts	*Percentage*
Roots	26.6
Leaves	5.8
Flowers	5.2
Fruits	10.3
Seeds	6.6
Stem	5.5
Wood	2.8
Whole Plant	16.3
Rhizome	4.4

Source : FRLHT.

Any Strategy should maintain the long-term view. In principle at least, medicinal plants could contribute substantially to the overall management of natural resources. Indeed, if given research and policy support, they could potentially become high-value components of many agriculture and rural development programmes, perhaps providing upscale alternatives to low-value food crops.

Cultivation

At present, the farming of medicinal plants is small, scattered, and largely informal. Given the increasing global population and consequent rise in demand for medicinal plants, one strategy option is to regard medicinally important species as underutilised crops.

Farming these species is not only an alternative to collecting plants from nature; it could help conserve the wild types by relieving some of the pressure on them. Cultivation also permits production of uniform material from which standardised products can be consistently obtained.

Cultivation should be a major part of any strategy. An increasing number of developing countries are already showing an interest in farming medicinal plants-trees, shrubs, lianas and herbs, annuals as well as perennials.

In principle at least, it seems possible that; he cultivation of medicinal plants could be appropriately included in many agricultural and rural development projects. It will demand social acceptance, the incorporation of indigenous knowledge, and farmer and community participation, but it cam be done.

The cultivation of medicinal plants provides opportunities for genetic improvement. For one thing, selection and vegetative propagation could produce cultivators that are rich in active ingredients and also have desirable agronomic traits such as good yields, pest and disease resistance, and environmental tolerance.

A well-managed cultivation programme presents an opportunity for local and national authorities as well as communities to exercise a beneficial influence over commerce in medicinal plants and their derivaties-a process that could guarantee both safety and efficacy and also ensure fair prices to collectors and cultivators. Both in-situ and ex-situ cultivation programmes could be promoted especially to protect those rare, endangered and vulnerable species most threatened in their natural habitats.

Investigations should be made into the stability of each herbal product, taking into account such practices as the effects of sunlight, temperature, humidity, plant husbandry, and packaging. But cultivation may also exacerbate environmental problems.

Pesticides and fertilise rs, for instance, represent a risk if indiscriminately used. In the United Kingdom, there is even now a proposal to produce 20,000 tons of daffodil bulbs annually for galanthamine, a product thought to slow the progress of Alzheimer's disease. Such large-scale production implies monocropping, perhaps with accompanying pest problems and a possible need of pesticides.

Table 3.8. Prices of Important Medicinal Plants in Madhya Pradesh and Delhi Markets (All figures in Rs./kg.)

Species	*Local Name*	*Katni*	*Jabalpur*	*Delhi*
		Price	*Price*	*Price*
Emblica officinalis	Aonla	800	140	600
Terminalia belerica	Bahera	90	200	250
Chlorophytum tuberosum	Safed musli, Kulai	14,000	25,000	20,000
Curcuma angustifolia	Tikhur	2,000	-	-
Embelia tsjeriam	Baybirang	800	-	-

Species	*Local Name*	*Katni*	*Jabalpur*	*Delhi*
		Price	*Price*	*Price*
Acorus calamus	Bach	1,200	900	-
Dioscorea daemona	Baichandi	1,100	-	-
Semecarpus anacardium	Bhilwa	100	100	500
Cyperus rotundus	Nagamotham, Mutha	200	900	-
Swertia chirayita	Chirayata	400	-	700
Woodflorida floribunda	Dhawi Phool, Dhua	200	-	700
Aegle marmelos	Bel guda	225	-	500
Rauwolfia serpentina	Sarpagandha	-	2500	6000

Certification for Raw Materials

Today, many of the medicinal plants available in the market place, are adulterated and are microbial contaminated. This is due to absence of raw-material certification requirements, for the industry by the FDA and absence of suitable post-harvest technologies, especially related to drying of medicinal plants. It is absolutely essential that ISM (Indian System and Medicines) Department sponsors and promotes regional certification facilities to set gold standards for raw drugs.

Initially, however, certification need not be made not be made compulsory. An agmark or ISO-9000 like standard for medicinal plants can be immediately promoted by the ISM Department, to encourage quality awareness in industry and amongst consumers.

The ISM Department can also support consumer research and education organisation to undertake consumer awareness campaign based on quality assessment of raw materials and finished products, used by the herbal industry.

Issues

- A valid methodology for certification of medicinal plants
- Mechanisms required to operationalise this

Quality Control

There is increasing concern regarding the quality of medicinal plant material being delivered to local pharmaceutical industries and the length of storage prior to processing. The storage time is of particular concern because of loss of efficacy. Any future strategy should encourage better handling and prompt deliveries. Therapeutic products from plants differ crucially in one particular aspect from those from a laboratory they are subject to the vagaries of nature.

National Coordination Mechanism

A national medicinal plants council, commission or board which can involve environment, health, science and technology, agriculture commerce ministries, the private sector and banks should be seriously considered as a mechanism to coordinate policy and administrative measures in this sector, that will (a) kick-start extensive cultivation (b) promote in situ conservation of genetic resources (c) promote gold standards for raw materials (d) regulate, and where it proves necessary, ban wild collections.

Issues

- The role of the Medicinal Plant Board in the regard.

Sustainable Bio-Partnerships

Commercialisation of the medicinal plant sector as it stands as it stands now is unplanned, unmonitored, poorly understood, grossly inequitable and opaque. What is needed is a process fully participated by all the major actors, down streamed to the lowest possible level in the production-to-consumption and marketing (PCM) continuum and equitable, ensuring fair benefits to the local people, specially the collectors.

The process of globalisation which has also started adversely impacting the micro economies of the sub sector, has added to the additional pressure to the on going commercialisation process which need to be constantly monitored, evaluated and managed.

However, increasing commercialisation of medicinal plants does provide opportunities to the local communities to enhance their livelihoods. But in order to realise this potential we need first to create a level playing field for all the players and stakeholders in the PCM continuum and ensure that the resources especially market information are made available to all the players. It is argued that this is possible in a framework of bio-partnership.

Table 3.9. Some of the Major Commercial Cultivation Areas of Medicinal and Aromatic Plants in India

Sl. No.	*Crop*	*Areas (ha)*	*States where grown*
1.	Psyllium (Plantago)	50,000	North Gujarat and Northwest Rajasthan
2.	Senna (Cassia)	10,000	Coastal districts of Tamil Nadu
3.	Opium poppy	18,000	Madhya Pradesh Rajasthan and Uttar Pradesh
4.	Asgand, Aswagandah	4,000	Central Parts of Madhya Pradesh
5.	Cinchona	6,000-8,000	Dajeeling district (West Bengal) Ootacamund district (Tamil Nadu)
6.	Ipecac	100	Northern West Bengal
7.	Khasi Kateri (Solanum viarum)	3,000	Maharashtra
8.	Japanese Mint	10,000	Uttar Pradesh and Punjab
9.	Basil	500	Uttar Pradesh
10.	Aniseed	3,000-5,000	Punjab and Western Uttar Pradesh
11.	Lemon grass	20,000	Kerala
12.	Palmarosa grass	2,000	Uttar Pradesh, Karnataka
13.	Citronella grass	2,000	Assam, Meghalaya, Andhra Pradesh
14.	Vetiver	Scattered	Kerala, Karnataka, Tamil Nadu
15.	Jasmine	2,000	Tamil Nadu, Karnataka
16.	Rose geranium	1,000	Tamil Nadu, Karnataka
17.	Damask	3,000	Uttar Pradesh

Policy and Regulations

Any nation's strategy for medicinal plant development needs to consider both current and potential in the future policies and regulations. Among points each nation needs address are:

- Is the use of medicinal plants encouraged in healthcare programs?
- Are there policies for conserving medicinal plants and incentives to encourage local community participation?
- Is there a policy for restoring plants harvested in the wild?
- Are there a policy for collectors and farmers to keep the production of medicinal plant?
- Does the government support research into these plants?
- What are the policies regarding the export of medicinal plants?
- Are only raw materials exported?
- Is "In-country" processing (which may further help the trade in medicinal plants)

Topics that Require in-depth Studies are

1. Current Status of Medicinal Plants

- Trade and Economics: so far no concrete data available on these aspects
- Status of medicinal plants in cultivation or wild also not available
- Links to modern medicine
- Links to biodiversity
- Links to agriculture (good, bad, and misrepresented)
- Links to forestry
- Medically useful wild plants
- Chemical synthesis and its relation to medicinal plants

2. Future needs for Medicinal Plants

- Genes to maintain productivity
- Potential for dramatic advances
- Changing opportunities (new market, new nutritional or health findings, etc.)

3. Threats to Medicinal-Plant Biodiversity

- Current losses of genetic diversity in medicinal plants
- Threatened wild varieties.

Table 3.9. Some practitioners of folk traditional medicines in South India

Traditional Carrier	*Subjects*	*Number*
Housewives and mothers	Home remedies; food and nutrition Millions	
Traditional birth attendants	Normal deliveries	700,000
Herbal healers	Common ailments	300,000
Bone setters	Orthopaedics	60,000
Visha Vaidhyas	Natural poisons	60,000
Other specialists	Skin, respiratory, mental illnesses, arthritis, dental, wounds, liver, fistula, piles	About 1 per 300 herbal Healers

4. Protecting Medicinal-Plant Biodiversity

- Preserving wild genes
- In-situ conservation
- Preserving by utilizing
- Ex-situ cultivation, conservation

5. Operational Issues

- Economic issues
- Policy issues
- Regulatory issues

6. Social Issues

- Medicinal plants in traditional systems
- Developing medicinal crops without losing their biodiversity and traditions
- Encouraging use (and preservation) of traditional medicines, practices, and knowledge.

- Enhancing social capital Trust emboided in the traditional healers; their herbal cures.
- Income generation.
- Values and constraints not well understood.
- What are required: policies, incentives, regulatory framework research support, market support, market information.
- Initiative to establish a network of herbal products research and training centres of excellence in both public and private sector; linked collaboratively to international institutions.
- Product development, clinical evaluation and horticultural research will be priority areas.

Table 3.10. Collection Charges of Medicinal Plants (MFP) in South India

Medicinal Plant	*Rs. / kg of fresh weight*
Phyllanthes emblica	3.00
Coscinum fenestratum	12.50
Curcuma longa	15
Stereospemum sp.	60
Desmodium gangeticum	2.50
Sida rhombifolia	2.00
Terminalia chebula	4.00
Strobinalia chebula	4.00
Hemidesmus indicus	30.00

Source : Muraleedharanetal, 1998.

Table 3.11. Economic Returns of Cultivated Species in Amarkantak Region, Madhya Pradesh

Species	*Yield (kg / ha)*	*Market Rate (Rs. / kg.)*	*Market Values (Rs.)*	*Total Expenses (Rs.)*	*Net Return (Rs.)*
Curcuma angustifolia	9800	6.00	58,800	10,760	48,040
Rauwolfia serpentina	850	75.00	63,750	9,480	54,270
Acorus calamus	3500	10.00	35,000	7,950	27,040
Chlorophytum tuberosum	150	150.00	25,500	9,480	13,020

Source : Goswami and Bhatnagar (1991).

Export credit, export promotion activities, tax rebate, brand building are some of the activities required to be taken up immediately to promote medicinal plant product export.

Developing the export market would require innovative measures. There is imperative need to consolidate mobilise , There is imperative need to consolidate mobilise , and organise the medicinal plant sector.

The world would look to India as a source of supply; and for India, global market is almost given. While India has the knowledge, skill and resource, it has neglected the opportunities in the global market. We have to gear up to face the challenges given by China and Korea in the sector. Industry needs to focus on exportable packages and services.

Organisational Set Up

The apex body of the Board is headed by the Union Minister of health and Family Welfare as Chairperson and Union Minister of State for Health and Family Welfare as Vice-Chairperson and other members are as follows:

Ex-Officio members: (i) Secretary, Department of India Systems of Medicine and Homeopathy; (ii) Secretary, Minister of Environment and Forests; (iii) Secretary, Department of Scientific and Industrial and Research; (iv) Secretary, Department of Bio-Technology; (v) Secretary, Department of Science and Technology; (vi) Secretary, Department of Commerce; (vii) Secretary, Department of Industrial Policy and Promotion; (viii) Secretary, Department of Expenditure; (ix) Secretary, Department of Agriculture and Co-operation; (x) Secretary, Department of Agricultural Research and Education; and (xi) Secretary, Ministry of Tribal Affairs.

Four nominated members: Having expertise in the field of (i) Medico-ethno botany; (ii) Pharmaceuticals Industry of ISM; (iii) Marketing and Trade; (iv) Legal matters and Patents.

Four nominated members representing exporters of : (i) ISM and H drugs; (ii) NGOs; (iii) Growers of medicinal plants; (iv) Research and Developments Industry groups.

Two nominated members representing: Federations Co-operatives dealing with medicinal plants.

One members from: Research Councils of Department of – (i) Indian Systems of Medicine and Homeopathy, (ii) Pharmacopoeial Laboratory of Indian Medicines/Homeopathic Pharmacopoeia

Laboratory, Ghaziabad, and (iii) two members representing State Governments (by rotation every two years).

Chief Executive Officer in the rank of joint Secretary as Member – Secretary.

MARKET SCENARIO OF MEDICINAL PLANTS

Domestic Scenario

Medicinal plants market in the country is today unorganised due to several problems. Medicinal plants are a living resource, exhaustible if overused and sustainable if overused and sustainable if used with care and wisdom. At present 95 per cent collection of medicinal plants is from the wild. Current practices of harvesting are unsustainable and many studies have highlighted depletion of resource base. Many studies have confirmed that pharmaceutical companies are also responsible for inefficient, imperfect, informal and opportunistic marketing of medicinal plants. There is a vast, secretive and largely unregulated trade in medicinal plants, mainly from the wild, which confusion to grow in the absence of serious policy attention with environmental planning. Confusion also exists in the identification of plant materials where the origin of a particular drug is assigned to more than one plant, due to which, adulteration in such cases. All these affect the market both directly and indirectly.

Marketing is a daunting problem, which affect the development of the plant-based industry in developing countries. Marketability of products will be a crucial factor in determining the failure or success of this sector. The market outlets can be for local use and for export. As for local use some products could reach the consumer directly while others have to be either further processed or used as secondary components in other industrial products. A clear understanding of both the supply-side issues and the factors driving the demand and size of the medicinal plants market is a vital step towards planning for both the conservation and sustainable use of the habitats of these plants as well as for ensuring continued availability of the basic ingredients used to address the health needs of the majority of the world's population.

Brief Global Scenario

According to the report of the World Health Organisation (WHO), a large population of the world relies on the traditional systems of medicines, largely plant based to meet their primary health care needs. India at present exports herbal materials and medicines to the tune of Rs.446 crores only while on has been estimated that this can be raised to Rs.3000 crores by 2005. The Chinese export based on plants including raw drugs, therapeutics and other is estimated to be around Rs.18,000- Rs. 22,000 crores. In view of the innate Indian strengths which interalia include diverse eco-systems, technical and farming capacity and a strong manufacturing sector, the medicinal plants area can become a huge export opportunity after fulfilling domestic needs.

Export: A part from requirement of medicinal plants for internal consumption, India exports crude drugs mainly to developed countries, viz. USA, Germany, France, Switzerland, UK and Japan, who share between them 75 to 80 per cent of the total export of crude drugs from India. The principal herbal drugs that have been finding a good market in foreign countries are Aconite, Aloe, Belladona, Acorus, Cinchona, Cassia tora, Digitalis, Ephedra, Plantago (Isabgol), Cassia (Senna) etc.

Source: Planning Commission – Task Force Report, 2000.

PROMOTIONAL AND COMMERCIAL SCHEMES

DESIGNATED AREAS FOR FINANCIAL SUPPORT

Project Proposals could be submitted in the following designated areas of promotional/Commercial schemes for overall development of medicinal plants in general and with special reference to 32 species, prioritised and identified by the Board viz:

1.	*Amla*	Emblica officinalis *Gaertn*
2.	*Ashok*	Saraca asoca *(Roxb.) de Wilde*
3.	*Ashwagandha*	Withania somnifera *(Linn.) Dunal*
4.	*Atees*	Aconitum heterophyllum *Wall. Ex Royle*
5.	*Bael*	Aegle marmelos *(Linn) Corr.*
6.	*Bhumi amlaki*	Phyllanthus amarus *Schum and Thonn.*
7.	*Brahmi*	Bacopa monnieri *(L.) Pennell*
8.	*Chandan*	Santalum album *Linn.*
9.	*Chirata*	Swertia chirata *Buch-Ham.*
10.	*Daruhaldi*	Berberis aristata *DC.*
11.	*Giloe*	Tinospora cordifolia Miers.
12.	*Gudmar*	Gymnema sylvestre *R. Br.*
13.	*Guggal*	Commiphora wightii *(Arn.) Bhandari*
14.	*Isabgol*	Plantago ovata *Forsk.*
15.	*Jatamansi*	Nardostachys jatamansi *DC.*

16. *Kalihari* Gloriosa superba *Linn.*
17. *Kalmegh* Andrographis paniculata *Wall. Ex Nees*
18. *Kesar* Crocus sativus *Linn.*
19. *Kokum* Garcinia indica Chois.
20. *Kuth* Saussurea costus *C. B. Clarke* (S.lappa)
21. *Kutki* Picrorhiza kurroa *Benth ex Royle*
22. *Makoy* Solanum nigrum *Linn.*
23. *Mulethi* Glycyrrhiza glabra *Linn.*
24. *Safaid Musali* Chlorophytum borivillianum *Sant.*
25. *Pather Chur* Coleus barbatus *Benth.*
26. *Pippali* Piper longum *Linn.*
27. *Sarpgandha* Rauwolfia serpentina *Benth. ex Kurz*
28. *Senna* Cassia angustinafolia *Vahl.*
29. *Shatavari* Asparagus racemosus *Willd.*
30. *Tulsi* Ocimum sanctum *Linn.*
31. *Vai Vidang* Embelia ribes Burm. f.
32. *Vatsnabh* Aconitum ferox *Wall.*

Proposals could also be taken up for any other medicinal plant for which there is assured market.

PROJECT PROPOSALS CAN BE SUBMITTED IN THE FOLLOWING AREAS

I. PROMOTIONAL SCHEMES

1. Survey and Inventorisation of medicinal plants.
2. In-situ *conservation and* ex-situ *cultivation plants.*

To encourage in-situ *conservation and* ex-situ *cultivation of selected medicinal plants, particularly endangered species which have appeared in Indian Red Data Book (IRDB) and negative list of CITES.*

- To create region-wise and species-wise medicinal plants demonstration centers (herbal gardens).

3. Production of quality planting material
   - To produce germ plasms of quality planting materials in bulk by developing improved agro-techniques and other appropriate technology.
4. Extension activities- Information, education and communication:

- Awareness through audio- visual aids, talks, training, workshops etc.
- Training and visit of growers and collectors to demonstrations plots, research centers and other related organisations in the country.

TASK FORCE ON CONSERVATION AND SUSTAINABLE USE OF MEDICINAL PLANTS

(i) "Health for All" continues to be a distant dream for India. With the increase in life expectancy and the problems of over crowding, air and water pollution, degenerative disease stress, allergies, diabetes, rheumatic and arthritic conditions, neurological conditions, memory disorders are likely to grow. Currently, about 85 per cent of women are anaemic on account of iron deficiency and 2.2 million children are afflicted with cretinism while another 6.5 million are mildly retarded. About 1.1 lakh women die every year of causes related to pregnancy and childbirth. This can affect the quality of life, productivity and the well-being of future generations. The health of women is especially important because if children are born to sick mothers, there will be problems in their later life.

(ii) Our per capita annual consumption of drugs of Rs.125 is the lowest in the world mainly because medicinal plants constitute the principal health care resources for the majority of population. The World Health Organisation (WHO) estimated that 80 per cent of the population of developing countries rely on traditional medicines, mostly plant drugs, for their primary health care needs. Also, modern pharmacopoeia still contains at least 25 per cent drugs derived from plants and many other, which are synthetic analogues built on prototype compounds, isolated from plants. Transition from synthetic drugs and microbially produced antibiotics to plant based drugs is rapidly gaining acceptance. Global resurgence in the use of plant based drugs is an opportunity for India to attain self-reliance and boost the export of herbal drugs.

(iii) The demand on plant based therapeutics is increasing in both developing and developed countries due to the growing recognition that they are natural products, being non-narcotic, having no side-effects, easily available at affordable prices and sometimes the only source of health care available to the poor. Medicinal plants sector has traditionally occupied an important position in the socio-cultural, spiritual and medicinal arena of rural and tribal lives of India. The global thrust areas for drugs from medicinal plants include disease conditions, whose incidence is increasing and where the modern drugs are either unavailable or unsatisfactory.

(iv) In a wider context, there is a growing demand for plant-based medicines, medicines, health products, pharmaceuticals, food supplements, cosmetics, etc., in the national and international markets. Conservation and sustainable use of medicinal plants are issues on which immediate focus is required in the context of conserving biodiversity and promoting and maintaining the health of local communities, besides generating productive employment for the poor with the objective of poverty alleviation in tribal and rural areas.

(v) International market of medicinal plants is over US $ 60 billion per year, which is growing at the rate of 7 per cent. India at present exports herbal material and medicines to the tune of Rs. 446.3 crores only which can be raised to Rs. 3,000 crores by 2005. China and India are two great producers of medicinal plants having more than 40 per cent of global biodiversity. China, besides meeting its domestic requirement is earning US $ 5 billion per year from herbal trade. There is thus an enormous scope for India also to emerge as a major player in the global herbal product based medicines. However, this requires a grand strategic plan, which takes a holistic of the entire situation to boost the export of Rs.10,000 crores by 2010 and minimising the import.

(vi) Medicinal plants are used at the household level in a self-help mode. One and a half million practitioners of ISM and H use medicinal plants in preventive/promotive and curative applications. There are about 4,60,000 registered practitioners of ISM and H using medicinal plants in the codified streams. Further, there are 7843 registered pharmacies of ISM and 851 of homeopathy and a number of unlicensed small-scale units.

(vii) At present, 90 per cent collection of medicinal plants is from the wild, generating about 40 million mandays employment (part and full) and since 70 per cent of plants collections involve destructive harvesting many plants are endangered or vulnerable or threatened. Currently medicinal plants are collected without paying attention to the stage of maturity. They are stored haphazardly for long period of time under unsuitable conditions. This results in deterioration in quality. Such materials are not acceptable to importers and standard manufacturing drug units.

(viii) Marketing of medicinal plants is inefficient, informal, secretive and opportunistic. As a result, the raw material supply situation is shaky, unsustainable and exploitative. This results in depletion of resource base, exploitation of rural people (who are the real stewards of the resource), adulteration and non-availability of quality herbal drugs for domestic consumption as well as for exports.

(ix) As the price paid to the gatherers tends to be very low, they often "mine" the plants, as their main objective is to generate income. A critical factor in wild harvesting is the availability of cheap labour to undertake the very labour intensive work of herbal gathering. Women are the main gatherers and also the users. With the rampant deforestation, women have to cover greater distances for the collection of herbs that once grew almost outside their habitation. As forest disappear and over harvesting for commercial use reduces the stocks of wild medicinal plant material, there is a corresponding drop in the availability of the plants normally used as the first and last resort for all health care by rural population.

(x) Despite the wealth of resources (biological, human and financial) available, the sector has not developed in the absence of absence of suitable standardisation, quality control and efficacy of drugs. It has yet to formalise and organise marketing and trade and integrate the development of medicinal plants from production to consumption to boost export of herbal formulations.

(xi) Medicinal plants sector has a number of stakeholders having divergent interests. Each stakeholder is interested in strengthening aspects of his sector only and ignoring the overall development. Unless coordinated efforts are made the sector cannot develop.

(xii) Several constraints exist due to inadequate awareness; inadequate investments in research and development; manufacturer – exporter dissonance; lake of quality and standardisation norms; and lack of adequate marketing and trade informations.

(xiii) The emergence of the new intellectual property regime in the light of India's joining WTO will pose important challenges in this sector. The task force recommended several actions that were needed on the part of the government, institutions, etc. to strengthen India's capacity in the protection of its intellectual property rights. In particular, creating digital databases of India's traditional knowledge was recommended as a priority activity to provide the evidence of this knowledge in the public domain as well as India's ownership of the knowledge. Modernisation of the Patent office and the Trade Mark Register is long overdue. R and D institutions have to maximise their patenting efforts.

(xiv) The Task Force recognises that apart from the software industry, the pharmaceutical sector is the only one showing a constant growth of 15 per cent and more. Medicinal plants can be viewed as a possible bridge between sustainable economic development, affordable health care and conservation of vital biodiversity. For sustainable and equitable development of the sector, the task force recommends the following programmes:

- Establishment of 200 Medicinal Plant Conservation Areas (MPCA), covering all ecosystems, forest types and subtypes preferably inside the protected areas already notified under the Wildlife Act.
- Medicinal plant species which are rare or endangered or threatened should be identified and their ex-situ conservation, may be attempted in the established gardens, plantations and other areas.
- Three gene banks created with the financial assistance of Department of Biotechnology should properly store the germplasm of all medicinal plants.
- Two hundred "Vanaspati Van" may be established in degraded forest areas (with an area of about 3500 – 5000 hectares each). Intensive production of medicinal plants from these "Vanaspati Vans" will produce quality herbal products and generate productive employment to 50 lakh people, specially women, who are skilled in herbal production, collection and utilisation. "Vanaspati Van" should be manged under JFM for benefit sharing to atercate poverty of tribals.
- One million hectares of forest area rich in medicinal plants (about 5000 hectares each at 200 places) should be identified, their management plans formulated and sustainable harvesting encouraged preferably under the JFM system. Such areas, besides producing herbal

products will generate employment for 50 lakh tribals on sustained basis and greatly help to alleviate poverty.

- Apart from CSIR, ICAR and ICFRE institution's engaged in medicinal plants about 50 NGOs, technically qualified, should be entrusted the job of improving awareness and availability of planting stock and agro-techniques for cultivation of medicinal. As recommended Twentyfive species having the maximum demand should be cultivated under captive and organic farming.
- All attempts should be made for medicinal plants screening/testing/clinical evaluation/safety regulation as well as research and development. Safety, efficacy, quality control, pharmacopoeia development should be expedited and completed by 2003.
- Policy, legal and institutional supports should be extended to the sector for adopting standards, quality control, efficacy and effectiveness of herbal drugs.
- Drug Testing Laboratories for ISM and H products should be established with qualified staff to test the plant/mineral based products. Training should be imparted staff, drug inspectors and to the quality control managers/in-charges of the manufacturing units so that they are able to identify the raw-materials for the presence of essential properties of medicinal plants.
- To prevent patenting of our traditional knowledge by outsiders, all the available information should be properly formatted in a digital from by using international standards for wider use both at the national and international level. Efforts should be intensified to create an Indian Traditional Knowledge Base Digital Library.
- The Task Force strongly recommends establishment of "Medicinal Plant Board" for an integrated development of the medicinal plants sector. It is expected to formalise and organise medicinal plants marketing and trade, coordinate efforts of all the stakeholders of the sector and ensure health for all by improving the awakening and availability of herbal products, besides generating productive employment to 10 million tribals and women on a regular basis. The "Medicinal Plant Board" will need a financial assistance of Rs. 50 crores over a period of three years.
- Ten major medicinal plants identified for export should

be extensively studied and appropriate literature on every aspect of such plants may be made available in the world market.

- *Medicinal plants sector for its integrated development will need a financial assistance of Rs.1000 crores over a period of 5 years. Besides the national efforts external funding may be explored to ensure* "Health For All" *by 2005 itself.*

(B) MARKET POTENTIALS OF MEDICINAL PLANTS IN THE STATE OF JHARKHAND

Diseases are the basic problems to all the people in various levels of culture. During recent time the social and cultural factors have been accepted by all concerned as of specific importance in the field of medicine and public health programme. In the region of Chhotanagar it is believed that man, money, fruit, animals, vegetables and medicinal plants are the creation of bhagwan (God) as a major source for healthy living. Resource belonging to older generations have an altogether different concept of disease and treatment which may be one of the reason for POOR LEVEL OF MARKETING OF MEDICINAL PLANTS IN THE STATE OF JHARKHAND. For the most part villagers avoid preventive care. Thus guardian spirits guard. The people of Chhotanagpur in general. It is believed that both Maha Deva and Parwati stand is the heaven as father and mother and take much care about their children. Excepting a few there is a general belief that the diseases are caused not due to infection from surrounding rather these are effected by some supernatural causes. Majority of the people are unknown of the germ theory of disease within the family the members frequently eat from the some dish and usually they are not in the habit of using separate utensils. Generally the villagers try to look at their health problems through socio-cultural perspective rather than trying for a so-called scientific explanation. According to they, the diseases are the out come of fallowing reasons.[15]

(a) An act of a number of gods and goddesses;

(b) Effect of karma (deeds) in previous life;

(c) Action of planets and stars; and

(d) Evil spirits effect animals and mens both.

It in further believed by the villages of chhotanagpur that proper remedies of diseases are-OJHA, GUNIN, DAYNEE, SOKH A BABA, FAKIR, PIR, MAULBI.

Such performers are a visible part of village life and DIVINE CURE through gods prayer can give protection from diseases. There are a number of specific folk deities believed to have power in bringing sickness or of curing. For example SITALA is responsible for pox and while MANASA for snake bites. TARIKKHE is supported to look after the sickness of eyes. SHASTHI looks after the well being of the children.

However there are some herbs and plants of the state of chhotanagpur which are sold by the villagers in the local markets of all the district. The undernoted table show the names of herbs and plants used to sold in the local market.

Table 3.12

Sl.No.	*Name of herbs and plants of Jharkhand*
1.	Bel
2.	Babul
3.	Siris
4.	Lahsun
5.	Dhritkumari
6.	Sharifa
7.	Kadam
8.	Safedmusli
9.	Satawar
10.	Neem
11.	Baans
12.	Kachnar
13.	Punarva
14.	Sarson
15.	Pthar chur
16.	Adrak
17.	Amrud
18.	Mehendi
19.	Karanj
20.	Bada gokhru

Sl.No.	*Name of herbs and plants of Jharkhand*
21.	Har singhar
22.	Mangraila
23.	Kamal
24.	Shahtut
25.	Karaila
26.	Chuimui
27.	Pudina
28.	Bakain
29.	Aam
30.	Jtamashi
31.	Bantulsi
32.	Ratanjot
33.	Chameli
34.	Gurhul
35.	Surajmukhi
36.	Safeed hurhur
37.	Gurmarbuti
38.	Gamhar
39.	Kaith
40.	Dudhi
41.	Baibhring
42.	Rajdhatura
43.	Dhatura
44.	Shisam
45.	Motha
46.	Haridab
47.	Rohish ghas
48.	Haldi
49.	Kalimusli
50.	Jeera

Sl.No.	*Name of herbs and plants of Jharkhand*
51.	Sukhdarshan
52.	Lisoda
53.	Shankh pushpi
54.	Gugul
55.	Pathar chur
56.	Kundru
57.	Aprajita
58.	Pilahurhur
59.	Dalchini
60.	Tejpatta
61.	Behera
62.	Safedmusli
63.	Bathua
64.	Rat ki rani
65.	Balkangani
66.	Deodar
67.	Sadabahar
68.	Amaltas
69.	Papita
70.	Satawar
71.	Bhang
72.	Palash
73.	Kaner
74.	Kapas
75.	Khaksa
76.	Sagwan
77.	Indrjaw
78.	Kagji nebu
79.	Aswagandha

Sl.No.	*Name of herbs and plants of Jharkhand*
80.	Sinduar
81.	Gulbanafsh
82.	Kala jeera
83.	Jangli pyaj
84.	Methi
85.	Palwal
86.	Chotagokhru
87.	Amla
88.	Pilakaner
89.	Aasan
90.	Harre
91.	Neem
92.	Arjun
93.	Imli
94.	Genda
95.	Sahtut
96.	Chiraita
97.	Kuchla
98.	Palak sag
99.	Pipal
100.	Saal or sakhua
101.	Til
102.	Ashok
103.	Ritha
104.	Semal
105.	Gulab
106.	Arandi
107.	Sarpgandha
108.	Jawayeen
109.	Aasan
110.	Kurthi ka daal

The people engaged in the marketing of medical plants in the state of Jharkhand and Bihar are as under :

Table 3.13

Sl. No.	*Name and Address of the Firm*	*Name of the Herbs*	*Category*
1.	Aakruti Enterprises Limited Address: Sector 3-B, 435, Bokaro Steel City - 827 003, India	Suppliers of lemon grass, Palmarosa, alovera, gerinium and other herbs Manufacturers and exporters of herbs.	Traders
2.	Bless Remedies Private Limited Address: S. S. Complex, Nai Sarai, Ramgarh Cantt, Ranchi 829 122, India Phone: +(91)-(6553)-223720 Fax: + (91)-(6553)-225756 Jharkhand	Manufacturers and exporters of herbs.	Manufact-urers
3.	Jharkhand Herbal Address: Dindayal Nagar, Near Ranchi College, Ranchi - 834 008, India Phone: +(91)-(651)-2310744	Manufacturer and exporters of safed musli, gurmar, anantmul, bakas	Manufact-urers
4.	Monalisa Herbs Address: Flat No. 52-C, 7th Phase (North), Adarshnagar Sonari, Jamshedpur - 831011, India Phone: +(91)-(657)-2225627	Exporters of medicines from herbal extracts.	Exporters
5.	Monalisa Herbs Address: Flat No. 52-C, 7th Phase (North), Adarshnagar Sonari, Jamshedpur - 831011, India Phone: +(91)-(657)-2225627	Exporters of medicines from herbal extracts.	Exporters
6.	Atma Address: C-67, Gandhi Vihar, Anisabad, Patna - 800 002, India Phone: +(91)-(612)-2250608 Fax: +(91)-(612)-2223470	Exporters of medicines from herbal extracts.	Exporters

Sl. No.	*Name and Address of the Firm*	*Name of the Herbs*	*Category*
7.	Shree Baidyanath Ayurved Bhawan Ltd. Address: Baidyanath Bhawan Rd, Patna-800001 Phone: 353048-647	Sellers of safed musli, sarpgandha, ashwagandha, pippli, bach, satavar etc.	Trader
8.	Synergy International, Sherghati Address: Gola Bazar, Arya Steel Udyog, Sherghati, Gaya - 824 211, India Phone: +(91)-(0)-9835368275	Manufacturer of exporters of natural herbs. Ayurvedic products	Manufact urers

A number of Non-Government organisations (NGOs) working on medicinal plants and folk medicine in different parts of India have collected a lot of data while useful information has also been circulated by students working for doctorate in some universities. There is a need for further work is this area to cover all the crude drug materials used in the production on and distribution of drugs in India in general and the state of Jharkhand in particular. The information required for this purpose is about the source from where the raw material is available, present production if cultivated or range and pattern of distribution and areas with rich population if originating from the wild. This type of study, though laborious and time consuming, is never the less very useful. The present work includes market studies such as PROCUREMENT, CHANNELS OF SUPPLY etc. in India in general and the state of Jharkhand in particular. There is a great need of continuing this type of studies on plant raw materials, Medicinal plant with production, Profit, market share, new customers, turnover, cost reduction, service time and complaints at local, national and global level, to make awareness of modern technology is the areas of marketing of medicinal plants and to educate its short term and long term benefits and to access.[16] The degree of understanding of Indian companies to access of international markets in the field of Medicinal plants and their products, Finally there is a need to analyse quality perceptions of medicinal plants of the state of Jharkhand and to find out the ways and means for keeping promises on moral basis of both in Governmental and private sector.

Jharkhand is universally famous for forest rich tribal culture, beautiful hills, hillocks forest cover, peremial rivers, spring of very prisons minerals and areas. The main source of income of tribal for their livelihood is forest and agriculture. In forest products, non timber forest products which includes medicinal and herbal plant play very important role in the tribal economy.

Many tribals are collecting the herbal and medicinal plants from nearest forest and sell it is the local market at a very low price. There is no support price of difference herbal plants, due to this the collectors of medicinal and herbal plants are fully exploited by the middlemen similarly the tribal people don't know about its appropriate price.

Most of the medicinal and herbal plants are exported from this region due to lack of knowledge about its technology, as well as its market looking to the rich bidder sity in the region there is a need of systematic survey of available medicinal and herbal plants including identification uses, valuation etc. Considering the agro climatic and practices of herbal and medicinal plants involving local farmers. Bio-diversity Board should be established to conserve the bio-diversity of the state. The board should give medicines name, cultivation, marketing and export of herbal and medicinal plants. Looking to the side effects of modern allopathic medicines the whole world is attracted towards the herbal and Locally available other medicinal plants in last few decades. The demand for herbal medicines is increasing day by day not only in the villages but even in the urban societies.[17]

Jharkhand is dominated with forest and tribal population. Most of tribal community is fully dependent on herbal medicines surrounding their habitat since ages to popularises Jharkhand as herbal state following points are to be considered.[18]

IDENTIFICATION OF MEDICINAL PLANTS

In Jharkhand State some of the medicinal plants have been over utilised include, KATFALA, KARUKI, ATIBISH etc. Due to over exploitation plant population of important medicinals and herbal plants has been reducing day by day.

In future if appropriate efforts are not made some of the medicinal plants like ASHWA GANDHA, RASNA, ISABGOL, BHRIN, GRAJ etc. will be disappeared from the region of Jharkhand.

In the forests of Bastar there are some medicinal plants like SANDHANPARNI (Desmodium gangecticum) also come into dangerous position due to slackness of the government of Jharkhand in particular and the people of the region in general. Looking at the above facts there is need to survey and list the various medicinal plants available in the state, efforts should also be made to conserve the disappearing medicinal and herbal plants.

Cultivation of Medicinal Plants

In Jharkhand state there is wide scope of cultivation of medicinal and herbal plants. A wide verities of medicinal and herbal plants are available in dense forests of Kodarma, Chaibasa and Khunti.

On river banks of Suwarn Rekha important herbal and medicinal plants such as saukhpushp, Brahmi, Gorakhmundi etc. grow. At present the commercial cultivation of herbal and medicinal plants is very limited while the climate of the region is very much suitable for the cultivation of medicinal plants. The required imputes like seed, plant etc. Should be sold through co-operative and other institutions so that the cultivations and collector shared, get proper remunerative price of their products looking at availability of medicinal plants care should be taken to conserve these valuable resources in kitchen garden and forest by the local people. Further a bio-diversity board should be established which will give new direction to medicinal and herbal plants cultivation, marketing and exploitation.

Establishment of bio-diversity boards is essential for proper identification, uses, and conservation of medicinal plants. If the Govt. of Jharkhand properly manage the production and marketing of medicinal plants no doubt the state would prosper as herbal state. At the availability of medicinal plants care should be taken to conserve these valuable resources in kitchen garden and forest by the local people.

Collection Centres of Medicinal Plants

Jharkhand has vast potential of herbal plants and medicinal plants. However the marketing facilities are very poor, few shops are available is the cities who purchase and sale important medicinal plants parts at high rate.

Minor forest products trade and development co-operative federation collects Harra Bhaera, Sal Seed, Tendu Leave with the help of villagers at village level co-operative centres.

Establishment of Pharmaceutical Industry

Tribal community in the region know the various medicinal uses of different species like Bagchi, Hathjod, amaltash etc. Pharmaceutical industries should also be established in the region as per availability and production. Local practitioner (Vaidya) has knowledge of medicinal use of different medicinal plants parts. The Government of Jharkhand should come forward to popularise the local medicines.

Establishment of Bio-diversity Board

The culture of Jharkhand is linked with plants, herbs and sharp. However, the marketing facilities are very poor. Hence, BIO DIVERSITY BOARD should be established for the growth of marketing of Medicinal plants and their products.

Specific Reference to the State of Jharkhand[19]

The medicinal plant and their products have a very long history of being utilised and trade in the Jharkhand state. There are the three main stakeholders involved the industry the consumers and the primary produces /collectors of row materials.

The chotanagpur region is bestowed with a variety of natural sources which have been exploited by making since time immemorial. One of the major sectors of natural recourses in the region in "medicinal plants" can be seen in ancient as well as modern literature including those dealing with Ayurved Systems of medicine. It is the believed that out of over 256 species (*Source*: NMPB) of medicinal plants traditionally used in Jharkhand, more than 10 per cent species come from the chotanagpur region.

In recent years there has been a sudden rise in the demand of herbal and products and plant based drugs across the jharkhand. India resulting in the heavy exploiting Medicinal Plants. Uncontrolled and unscientific harvest of several species and habitat degradation.

Chotanagpur plateau and santhal praganas is very rich in forest wealth. Ranchi, the capital of the state have 25 per cent forest area having a very rich stock of medicinal Plants. The indigenous people which compromise about 70-75 per cent of the total population of district still 100 per cent day depend on indigenous herbal medicines for the treatment of all sorts of ailments/ disorders/ daises. A large number of Indigenous people although mostly illiterate are experts in Identifying there medicine to the venders. They depend totally on the profession for their livelihood. The venders are actually the stockiest of the raw medicinal plants and also the suppliers for the practitioners such as Kabirajs, Vidas, Pahas. There Practitioners use to sell these in the form of drug in the village hats and even from this houses they prepare drug by necessary to investigate their economics and the reason of their economic exploitation so that they could get maximum price of the valuable medicinal raw materials.

Distribution of Medicinal plants starting from the collectors point and ending to the consumers. The collectors sent Sufficient time in collection washing of the Material, Drying of the Materials and the get meager amount from the vendors. The Vendors usually do not purchase the raw materially in weight but in bundles measuring bowls and bunches. The prices mentioned in the Table-I have been taking a normal standard of sough for each material.

The table clearly shows the fact the earning of the collectors. As a Specific Materials increases varying from 375 per cent when it comes to the hand of consumers from the collectors.

The table also exhibits the fact the earning of the collectors is negligible in comparison to vendors and the practitioners. Further the study also makes clears the reason why the collectors are poor Actually they are being exploited their collection to them at a nominal price, The Practitioners also do not use to purchase directly from the collectors. Being stockiest the raw use are always available with vendors and such as the Practitioner do not purchase directly from the collectors because the collectors are always ready to supply.

The critical study has exploited a very significant exploitation of the poor collectors on one hand and also the practitioners on the other hand by the vendors. This alarming Situations need immediately attentions by the administration to establish registered system of making where by the collectors should get sufficient amount far the raw materials. This will check the exploitation being done by the vendors on one hand and it will certainly reduce the price of the drug on the other hand. Since there will be no exploitations in the form of vendors as the consumers will also feel comfortable.

For successful marketing of medicinal plants and products, the first and foremost task is to boost up the cultivation with uncompromising standard of quality.

In fact, Cultivation of medicinal plants is not so easy. It is rather a challenging task to procure suitable planting materials and propagating then Successful.

Quality of the Finished Products Depend Largely on[20]

1. *Seeds and propagation materials-* seeds or planting materials has to be certified so that the harvested products contain adequate quantity and quality of active ingredients.

2. *Cultivations* –Depending upon on the method of cultivating e.g. Conventional or organic grower should be allowed to follow. Different standard of operating Procedures far cultivation. In general care should be taken to avoid environmental disturbance. The principal of good crop husbandry must be followed in including an appropriate rotation of crops.
3. *Harvest* – Harvest should take place when the plants are of best possible quality, according to this different utilisation.
4. *Primary Processing* – Primary processing after harvesting includes such steps as washing, Freesing drying etc. All these processes whether far food or medicinal use, must conform to international standard.
5. *Packaging* – Primary processed items should be free from law quality and foreign bodies. The Products should be packed in clean and dry sacks or boxes.
6. *Storage and transport* – Package dried materials and essential oils should be stored in and dry well aerated building in which the daily temperature fluctuations are limited and good aeration is guaranteed. For Fumigation of warehouses trained personnel should use only permitted substances.
7. *Process equipment* – All the equipment used far primary and secondary processing should be of standard quality.
8. *Education* – It is highly advisable to educate all the personnel dealing with the crops as those engaged in management of production, in production techniques as well as appropriate use of herbals and pesticides.

In Jharkhand women are mainly the collectors of medicinal plants in rural areas. They would be encouraged to Participate in Personnel interviews based on standardised questioners and include queries in to types of plants collected from forests farms, genders as brought into the market. Following factors would be taken into consideration far reasons such as on traditional medicinal Plants.

1. Information on medicinal Plants.
2. Correct identification of plants.
3. Parts of medicinal plants used.
4. Proper Past harvest treatment and preparation from plant parts.
5. Types of plants harvested over the rainy season.

6. Availability or non- availability of the plant used i.e. whether the plant has become more difficult to find in recent years.
7. Most important plants used during the last one years period.
8. Types of medicinal plants to be conserved.
9. Types of plants harvest over the rainy season.
10. Age of Plant.
11. Demand of medicinal plants by various herbal industries and pharmacists.
12. Listing of different Medicinal Plants with references to major soil types in the region.

There are more than 7000 species of plants used far medicinal purposes by the people of India of which 400 species are found in Jharkhand. There are two main steams of medicinal Knowledge in Jharkhand. That local folk are medicine located in villages and codified knowledge systems in ayurveda and other farms.

It is almost importance to prepare an inventory of these 400 species of medicinal plants that have been used far centuries by traditional practitioners as herbal medicine. Electronic database are in vogue far documenting traditional knowledge. This type of Documentation facilitates the survival of oral knowledge and prevents erosion of social process that percolate the knowledge of a community or tribe to its next generation. Keeping all these in mind five database are being built up on the medicinal plant species of Jharkhand with this surge in document action of traditional Knowledge database would gain prominence and command high revenues.

Nomenclature Database : A plant is known by different names in different regions of the country. This database provides reliable cross linkages between local and traditional names used in medicinal literature and botanists hence can use botanical names and Hence can be used by botanists and also by layman. And their traditional knowledge physician this kind of information is indispensable if we ought to do any serious work on medicinal plant application in India. The Field in database include Local name, Botanical name cited in Literature, Name in Trade.

Herbarium Database : Jharkhand lacks a central facility in the form of reliable Herbarium. Herbarium special are valuable far proper identification of species Medicinal plant Species. Besides providing an image of the stored specimen in the herbarium, this database provides information on habitat, no. of duplicates threatened, statues, Medicinal Systems of use, biotic association of the plant data and place of collection local name, language etc.

Propagation Database : The availability of data pertaining to propagation methods and seed storage of medicinal plant is very rare kind information is scattered in various print and electronic media dealing with a wide range of subjects ranging from forestry agriculture horticulture and medicinal plants. In this data base attempts are being made to collect and compile information on propaganda method, best season, month of planting media, soil type, special treatment (if requirement) germination data and seed storage data.

Distribution Database and Eco-distribution Mapping : A computerised is being developed to incorporate a range of data on distribution as well as habit life form of medicinal plant of Jharkhand. The information would be base on collection and compilation of data on precise locations of presence/collection of each prioritised species from a variety of sources like herbarium collection, literature data (flora) and primary survey data will be used far mapping the distribution through precise latitude and longitude coordinates.

Raw Drug Database : Medicinal Plants are cultivated mainly for this drug content. The quality and quantity of the active principles within the plants and varies forms season to season and under different conditions. The stakeholders of medicinal plants cultivation must know the trade of the plants. The optimum condition under which the active principal of the plants are best retained and the forms at different stages of trade with cost. Information pertaining to all these aspects would being corporate into this data base. The main objectives of this study is to blend traditional knowledge with Scientific methods of essential far establishing a participatory adaptive management methodology far sustainable harvest of medicinal plant from nature.

Jharakhand a land of forest and minerals, which is also, called India's mineral and agricultural state. The state is full of forest and minerals. In that forest, the number of plants is available which is useful for traditional medicine.

In spite of tremendous development in the field of allopathic during 21st Century, Plants still remain as one of the major natural source of drugs in both in modern as well as traditional System of natural products especially plant derived drug have been discovered on the basis of traditional or local medical practices.

In recent times, due to increasing realisation of health hazards toxicity caused by Synthetic drugs, there has been a renewal of interest in the use of plant-based drugs through out the world. There is number of herbal plants are available in Jharkhand forest which have diverse uses as raw material not only for medicine but also for articles of daily uses like toothpastes, talcum powder, shampoos, soaps and even to the extent of bio-pesticides in the agriculture management practices. A campaign is being going on entire country to utilise more and more plant derived chemicals in the human health care/personal care System. On the other hand, the trade on herbs and herbal drugs is growing substantially. Some of the facts about herbal drugs are :

1. Nearly 300 years ago, No pharmaceutical medicine were there and around are lakhs medicinal Plant species were the main sources of herbal drugs for entire population of Country.
2. According to an estimate about 2/3rd of over population cannot afford western medicines.
3. Even in entire country, Prescribed drugs bear 25 per cent of one or more herbal ingredients.
4. According to an estimate, about 30-40 per cent Pharmaceutical preparation are obtained from higher plants only.

The Knowledge of herbal drugs throughout the Jharkhand state can be proved by the following facts.

Table 3.14

Region / Content	*Yearly Turnover (Rs. in Lakh)*	*Annual growth rate (approx)*
Hazaribagh	6500	8-9%
Patratu	500	15-16%
South-east Jharkhand	2600	12-14%

Source : Personal Survey.

Jharkhand can be the bio-diversity center of India with the help of different agro – climatic ones, vegetative zones, biotic provinces, hesitable for specific species.

Unfortunately, Systemic efforts to explore and exploit these wealth is meager within the state but momentum of wild collection from the forest and marketing's been going on since long more than 80 per cent of Indian medicinal plants are collected from 17000 hectares of forest.

Jharkhand's out of 400 plant species (15 per cent of market (approx) nearly 400 species are of medicinal plant value some species are endangered plant :

Curcuma Longta	Ferula asafetida
Gymnema Sylbestre	Rawwolfia serpentine
Acorus calamus	Curcuma Aromatica
Piper cubeba	Curcuma causes
Aristotelian indica	Curcuma yedoaira
Commiphora mukul	Dyscoria Floribunda
Glorious superba	Dyscoria alata
Plumbago rosea	

CRUDE HERBAL DRUG

Jharkhand, being one of the market I in India, is also the center of big crude drug dealers in Eastern Region.

On the basis of demand of these crude drugs, the dealers trade the following crude herbs.

Table 3.15

(a) Sarpagandha	(Roulfia serpentina)
(b) Aswagandha	(withania somnibera)
(c) Kelmegh	(Andrographic paniculate)
(d) Sonapatta	(cassia angustifolia)
(e) Bael	(Bacopa monnieri)
(f) Baofl	(Bacopa monnieri)
(g) Amla	(Emblica officinalis)
(h) Haritoki	(Terminalia clebula)
(i) Jaipal	(Myristicaf ragruns)
(j) Pipul	(Piper Longum)
(k) Neem	(Ayadirachta indica)
(l) Jastimadhu	(Ghycyrrhiyu)
(m) Bahera	(Terminalia bellirica)
(n) Mesorshingi	
(o) Natakarajay	
(p) Jatamanishi	

Source : Personal Survey.

The quantity of crude drug brought from single shopkeepers per month and the price of respective crude drugs are :

Table 3.16

Name	*Price / kg (approx)*	*Quantity*
(a) Aswagandha	30-60	80-120
(b) Kalmegh	8, 10, 12	300
(c) Sonapatta	12,13, 30	400
(d) Brahmi	5	100
(e) Amla	17, 12	200
(f) Bael	8, 10	40
(g) Bahera	2	300
(h) Haritoki	3	300
(i) Nata Karanjay	14, 20	200
(j) Mesorshingi	20, 30	200
(k) Jastimadhu	30, 40	250
(l) Jaipal	60, 100	300
(m) Jatamansi	70, 100	225
(n) Sapagandha	75	100-200
(o) Pipul	70 – 90	300
(p) Neem	5	200

Source : Personal Survey.

Market Analysis

Considering the above data's. The Total money transacted by single crude drug dealer is,

Table 3.17

Name	*Price / kg (approx)*	*Quantity*
(a) Aswagandha	30-60	80-120
(b) Kalmegh	8, 10, 12	300
(c) Sonapatta	12,13, 30	400
(d) Brahmi	5	100

Name	*Price / kg (approx)*	*Quantity*
(e) Amla	17, 12	200
(f) Bael	8, 10	40
(g) Bahera	2	300
(h) Haritoki	3	300
(i) Nata Karanjay	14, 20	200
(j) Mesorshingi	20,30	200
(k) Jastimadhu	30, 40	250
(l) Jaipal	60,100	300
(m) Jatamansi	70, 100	225
(n) Sapagandha	75	100-200
(o) Pipul	70 – 90	300
(p) Neem	5	200

BAZAR MEDICINE - FLOATING HERBAL DRUG

People particularly from Village and Sub urban region are Optimistic. They use herbal medicine for the treatment of minor disease Collected from local market. Moreover, These people knows the traditional use of herbal drugs. These so called bazaar medicines, are being supplied by local market.

The Chief bazaar medicines traded in rural, Sub urban, urban and City. Areas are given:

Table 3.18

(a)	Shetbarela	(Sida rombifolia)
(b)	Bilbo	(Aegle marmelos)
(c)	Anantamul	(Hemidesmus indicus)
(d)	Bamonhati	(Derodendnon indicum)
(e)	Aswagandha	(Withania Somnifera)
(f)	Ayapang	(Eupatorium ayapana)
(g)	Boncharal	(Desmodium gyrens)
(h)	Lajyaboti	(Nimosa Pudica)
(i)	Khirikha	(Ghogfita)

The Demand of these drugs per month from a single big shop of state as a streat market is given below :-

Table 3.19

Name	*Demand (approx)*	*Price/kg (approx)*	*Total price*
Rambasak	0.8	80	100-150
Shatberela	0.3	60	80-110
Bilbo	4.5	15	220
Khrika	3	8	120
Ayapang	-	-	120
Bidyadarak	3	20	200
Bamonhati	2	8	120
Boncharal	-	-	200
Lajyapati	-	-	200

Total transaction of bazaar medicines from a Single market = Rs. 2000.

Basic, on 150% of above the real transaction of bazaar medicine per month from a single.

Market=3000* 100/15=20000.

Market Analysis of Jharkhand State.

(i) Transaction of bazaar medicines per month in the Ranchi City.

From a Single shop of a City=500

Market, Transacted money per month=700

Let, there are 10 shops in a city market

Money transacted=20000

In a City, there be 3 such shop which is located as there big shop thus Money Transacted=3000

(i) Transaction Of Bazaar medicines per month in and around city Sub-urbans.

Let, from a single town, money transacted per month from a Single town=Rs. 600

If there are at least 3 such shops in single town, then Money transacted=Rs. 3000=00

Let, there are 10 such base towns which is related with Marketing of medicinal Plant— Rs. 9000.

(ii) Transaction of Bazaar medicines around RURAL AREAS OF Jharkhand

Let from a Single shop in a single Village, money Transacted per month – around Rs. 1000.

If there are at least 3 villages around a single town,

Money transacted=Rs. 5000.

Thus, money transacted as bazaar medicine in and around Jharkhand district.

Rs. = 9000

Rs. = 3000

Rs. = 6000

Total Rs.= 18000

AROMATIC/ESSENTIAL OIL

Aromatic Plants have been of great interest to mankind from the beginning of human Civilisation. Aromatic Plants, and their products, Particularly the Essential oils are now becoming are of the more important export items. Essential oils are Chemical compounds with an odoriferous nature.[21]

Jharkhand has enjoyed a pre–eminent position in the manufacture of superior perfumes and aromatic by using essentials oils. In the India's Market it ranks 5th in position.

The chief essentials oil can be exported outside of the Jharkhand are :

(a) Japanese mint oil

(b) Kusum oil

(c) Karanj oil

(d) Lemongrass oil

(e) Palma Rosa oil

(f) Ginger oil

(g) Clove oil

(h) Eucalyptus oil

(i) Pepper oil

(j) Aaguri oil

(k) Vitiver oil

Herbal drug Industry is also Growing rapidly in the state of Jharkhand if they can find potential of Medicinal and Aromatic plants condition in this area.

The Dealers get these aromatic plants Particularly from the southern Jharkhand in a region of Western Ghats. The name of aromatic plants and their source as under :

(a) Lemon Grass Oil — Patratu, Southern Jharkhand
(b) Palmarosa Oil — Lathehar Southern Jharkhand
(c) Kusum Oil — Nagri
(d) Rose Oil — Southern Jharkhand
(e) Encalptus Oil — Southern Jharkhand
(f) Mint Oil — Palamu Jharkhand
(g) Karanj Oil — Latehar Jharkhand

The Market price of some of essential oil are as under:-

Name	*Rs per k.g. (approx)*
Lemon grass Oil	200
Karanj Oil	150
Palmarosa Oil	350
Mint Oil	150-300
Argundi Oil	20 –42
Rose Oil	6500
Kusum Oil	6000

A fraction of essential oil is also imported to India. The Names of essential oil and respective exporters are:-

(a) Lavander oil — France, Italy, alps.
(b) Lemon Oil — France, Italy, alps.
(c) Olive oil — Brazil Italy
(d) Orange oil — California
(e) Bargamolt Oil — California

Export potential of herbal Drug Market from Jharkhand.

There is growing demand for plant based medicines, health products, Pharmaceuticals, food supplements, cosmetics in Indian Market.

The international market of medicinal plant is over 60 billion US $ per year growing @ and P.A. The present export of herbal material and medicine is about Rs. 500 Crores. Other export of medicinal plant is china which export about per cent Billion US $ per year.

In India in Jharkhand Region total Value of Crude Drugs can be exported around 100000 Lakh (approx) in a year.

Herbal drug Industry is also Growing rapidly in the state of Jharkhand if they can find potential of Medicinal and Aromatic plants condition in this area.

In Jharkhand region based on the survey the present potential of herbal drug is 400 species and if it is properely exploited and marketed the potential for export can be to extent of 20 per cent to start.

MARKETING CHANNELS

Traders at the roadhead and along the main trails are the critical 1 link between medicinal plants and the market. They receive market information on species and price along with cash advances from large wholesalers from the plain, and they are the first major point of transaction for local collectors (Fig. 1). There

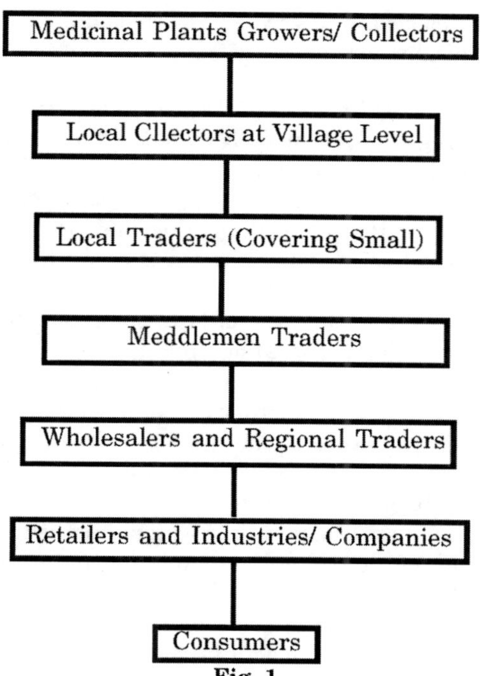

Fig. 1.

are many traders who double as shopkeepers, lodge operators, and farmers. In addition, a number of opportunistic buyers from plain or owners of firms periodically visit the region in search of more direct supplies.

Crude Herbal Drug

Jharkhand, being one of the market I in India, is also the center of big crude drug dealers in Eastern Region.[22]

Resident traders have their own territories based on kin relations or other historical ties. They are of different ethnicities and have varying levels of business savvy and political influence. At times they may work in collusion, but mostly operate independently. As such roadhead prices can be competitive, and a collector is free to sell as he please. Contrary to popular nations, the relationship between resident traders and collectors is not necessarily exploitative. Traders can play a very important role in village economices by providing a needed source of credit cash and marketing assistance. Traders and collectors may also be bound together by a mutually beneficial ritual brotherhood. On the other end of the scale, certain powerful traders may force collectors to sell exclusively to them. All these arrangements were observed in the buffer zone village and other villages located in higher altitudes areas of the Jharkhand.

Gaps in the Marketing Chain – the Black Hole

The marketing analysis usually ends at the community or perhaps the initial middleman. It is this part of marketing channel- after the product leaves the community or initial middleman and before its arrivals at the processor or the final consumer- which is relatively less is known, especially if the products are illegals, taxed, or regulation ban harvest or export. In order to fill in the gaps, current marketing analysis often estimates products (and income) flows by taking information obtained from a community and projecting it through a sequence of exchange until it reaches the final consumer, or taking information obtained from the retailer or processor and projecting it back to the collector (table 6.1),. This form of analysis may provide a rough estimate of the amount of the product in the marketing system, but it does not explain the processor of the marketing system (including who does the collection, level of household dependency on the product, sustainability of current harvest levels, and sharing of income and benefits, the important role of the middleman in providing cash advances, transport, or additional or preferred marketing channels of the product.

Barriers to Market Information

There are barriers to filling in the gaps between producers and the consumers or large processor. While the marketing channel can be determined, other information concerning the amount of the product, prices, and destination are more difficult to obtain. one of the primary barriers in obtaining information is the difficulty of gaining access to the major wholesalers or processor. Accuracy of information is also a problem and more difficult to ascertained. in village or the initial assembly points (i.e., the roadhead) observation combined with an interview can provide fairly accurate information. However, when interviewing (or attempting to interview) a wholesaler, the large quantity and variety of products on site may make verification of information difficult.

Regulations that encourage the flow of products into illegal channels also make it very difficult to do an accurate analysis. Information can be obtained on legal exports from official documents, although it should be recognised that products that are carried by porters across a border or region, the amount sold, benefits/income distribution etc., of what is not "formally" exported, but sold in local markets, or utilised by the local community is therefore based on estimates from case studies, and the 'bits and pieces' of information that are available.

Marketing and Sustainability

Information on the flow of products is important not only for marketing analysis, but also for an assessment of the sustainability of the market for medicinal plant cultivation and conservation. in order to determine sustainability, information must be gathered on current and past yield and marketing patterns, communities' perception of whether medicinal pkant resources are more or less prevalent than in the past, and the fuure market demand (Maikhuri et al. 2000a; Rao et al; 2002) external markets exert the greatest pressure on forest resources. Without external markets, communities utilise the resources, but there is little 'push' to gather/cultivate more of a product than can be utilised by the household or community. When marketing opportunities do appear, the community may have difficulty in cultivating the medicinal plants since they are facing problem in obtaining good quality and sufficient quantities of planting materials. They are also uncertain about the yields. Only few studies have reported the yields of medicinal plants and the cost : benefits ratios (table 2, maikhuri et. al. 2000b).

Control of Resources

While there might be traditional mechanisms to regulate, access and gather the forest products, these rights of control (including right of exclusion) are frequently no longer recognised by other communities who want access to the resources or by the state or state agencies. Local communities are often minorities with little political power. The communities right to live in or adjacent especially with the current global concern for conservation. When the income from a product incresease, then competition within a community and between communities may increase as well. Within the community, the dependency on forest products will be related to other resources of the household. It is common to find that it is the poorst households, with less agricultural land, livestock, adult females/males, etc. That are the predominant gatherers of forest products. While the actual amount of income earned from Non – Timber Forest Products may be small, it may provide the largest portion of that household's income. There are the households that are the most vulnerable to competition both within and among communities.

Valuation and Pricing Mechanism

There are few perfect markets. The predominant pattern in medicinal plants and other forest product markets is many producers, a small number of wholesalers or processors, thus rather than competition, cooperation among the wholesalers results. In medicinal plants and other forest products, the buyers usually sets the price and the gatherer/grower responds to the price. Theorectically, if the price for a products is regarded by the collector as being high (a good price), more will be cultivated / gathered and sold.

Total income of per hector production and price for various medicinal plants (In India) However, local communities often have few options for generating income. The lack of alternatives for income results in medicinal plants those cultivated or gathered sold even when price are relatively (based on price history for the product) low. It is this lack of alternatives that results in the low prices of medicinal plant and other forest products in many local communities.

There is a lack of information. The gather may know what the consumer wants or need. While products flow out, little information flow in. The longer the marketing chain, the less likely that this information will be available to the producer. the middlemen may not know what is desired by the final consumer and may not effectively get this information to the producer. Price information also many not flow back to the grower/ collector. Few collectors (or middlemen) may know the final price paid by the consumer or processor. While this may in some instances be intentional (in order to keep the profit at the other end of the marketing chain), it is also the result of the distance the product may travel as well as the lack of awarness that the current system may be changed. without this information it is difficult for a grower/ collector to determine what is a good price and the real value. Also, without information as to the value determined by what a customer is willing to pay for the product, the collector canot negotiate for a larger portion of the final price.

Marketing is the process of exploring which products potential customers will purchase and then producing, processing, promoting and distributing the products at a profit. In reality, the gatherers/ growers of Medicinal plants do not market their products, rather they sell the products to a customer (the middleman). If the goal is for the communities to to retain a larger portion of the income generated by medicinal plant cultivation the task of both producer and those involved in assisting market development of both the products is to transform the current process from selling to marketing at the community level. Howevere, there are obstacles inherent in medicinal plant growers/ gatherers and the current marketing system that will hinder this transformation (Box 1.)

Box I
Market and Marketing of Medicinal Plants: A Major Constraint

- Market for medicinal plants is very erratic and shows wide disparity in their market values.
- Barriers to information : Information concerning the amount of the product, price and destination is more difficult to obtain.
- Many other problems related to the marketing of medicinal plants :
  - (i) small quantities/many collectors,
  - (ii) services provided by middleman, and
  - (iii) policy and regulation.

To develop marketing systems that provide greater benefits to the community (and might lead to conservation of the species) the following is needed :

- (i) local management of medicinal plants
- (ii) cooperatives
- (iii) removal of regulations, and
- (iv) market analysis

Factors Influencing Prices

The prices of medicinal plants also show variations as per demand – supply scenario. besides, the price are also affected by the seasons and increased by the discovery of new drugs or medicinal properties of a particular plants. Taxus baccata leaves prices suddenly increased with discovery of the properties of palant for curing cancer. Similarly legal, illegal and unsustainable harvesting and use of valuable Medicinal plants affects their availability and thus increase the price.

Processing and Value Addition

Establishing processing and semi-processing units in the form of small cottage industries dealing with medicinal plants at the village level in the inaccessible, remote and far–flung areas would definitely ensure better profits to the primary growers or collectors. It will not only reduce the transportation and carriage expenses of raw materials but will also provide ample opportunities to generate wage employment for rural population. There measures to be incorporated in the category of semi-processing of the raw materials are cleaning and grading to be performed at the collectors/growers level which will not only enchance the price but also improve the quality of the material. Besides, the value addition of medicinal plants may involve activities like drying, pulping, making concentrates, powdering, boiling, distilling etc. which may be done at village or community level but it must ensure the quality of the final materials. The semi-processing and value addition at the grower/collector level might be suitable provided there is an assured buyback arrangement with an industry or exportes or big businessman. Even simple activities related to processing semi-processing and value addition medicinal plants are found difficult to managed by the poor farmers/colled. Therfore, those small processing and semi-processing units may run smoothly at village or community level which may provide viable returns to the people community involved in short-and long term basis.

Poilcy interventions for medicinal plant cultivation has to consider marketing as a major component and developing medicinal plant information bulletins similar to horticultural information bulletins to collect, compile and disseminate the production, processing and consumption of these low volume and high value crops. Such initiatives will required not only government mobilisation byt also participation of all stakeholders in the marketing chain in Jharkhand region.

Medicinal Plant Raw Material for Indian and Pharmaceutical Industry

Assessment of resources of medicnal plants raw mateial required by indian drug and pharmaceutical indusry indicates a high potential of further development through a comperhensive approach. However, There are number of problem which are to be tackled to obtain desired results. the country with a rich plant diversity, wide spectrum of agro -ecological conditions and advanced scientific and managerial expertise and infrastructure, lags behind many countries in this sphere. A serious potential is needed to identify weakness and stregth in this regard. The issues requiring immediate attention are discussed here.

Systematic Census and Invention

There is no inventorisation of medicinal plants at national level, the flora of India has been worked out in detail and inventories of palnts occuring in most parts of the country are available in various floras, compendiums and manuals. The country is dotted with a lage number of herbaria housing well preserved and identification plant specimens, most of which carry notes on distribution patterns flowering and fruiting period, local uses and other useful information. A lots of work has been carried out on medico-ethno botany by research councils working under department of Indian syatem of Medicine (ISM) and through certain projects sponsored by the Mininstry of Environment and Forest. Anumber of Non-Govt. Organisations (NGOs) working on medicinal in medicinal plants and folk medicine in different parts of india have collected a lot of data while useful information has also been collected by students working for doctorate in some universities. Systematic retrieval of relevant information from these source and its consolidation at a single place is highly desirable in making a proper assessment of medicinal plant resources of the country.

Identity of Botanical Source botenical identity of a majority of plants mentioned in the Pharmacopeia of 'Ayurvedic' 'Unani' and other traditional system of medicine practiced in India, has been located since the introduction of morden system of plant classification in the Satate of Jharkhand there, however, are a number of medicinal plant and crude drugs where the identity of plant source has not been finally established.

Among the medicinal plant and crude drug materials having more than one botanical source, those belonging to the species of the same genera and family do not pose much of a problem. In most of such cases, chemical composition is similar, though concentration of major constitues may differ. Thus, the three species of genus Berberis, sold in the market by the name of Daruharidra have berberine as major alkaloid. Its concentration is highest in the roots of berberis Chiritria.

The raw matrial used by drug and pharmaceutical industry is generally procured through market channels and are somethimes found adulterated pharmacognostic studies have been done for a number of important crude drug material to distinguish the genuine material from the adulterant. Such information has been recorded in various pharmacopoeias. Under the present pattern of utilisation, however, the material is obtained and processed in large quantities and use of such information is generally found impractical. the efficient way to determine adulteration is through morphological and organoleptic stuidies. Another method used for this purpose is thin layer chromatography (TLC) and high pressure liquid chromatograpghy which is employed for the analysis of extractives of the samples of the crudes drug, collected at random. On account of its rapidity and ease of visual evaluation, TLC finger-priting has become popular for identification of the plant source of the crude drug under use. This method can however, be employed only by a large manufactureres of drug who are able to establish these facilities. For others, the use of morphological and organoleptic characters will be the right tool for authentication purpose. The author has carried out studies on about 200 crude drug materials largely and regularly employed by the Indian drug and pharmaceutical industry (Sarin, 1996). there is a need for further work in this area to cover all the crude drug material useds in the production of drugs, pharmaceuticals cosmetic and other over the counter products.

Techno-Economic Evaluation

The informntion required for this purpose is abput the source frpom where the raw material is avlable; present productionb if cultivated or range and pattern of natural distribution and areas with rich poulation if orginating from the wild. The study of growth parsmeters in relation to ecological conditions prevailing in the areas where the plant grows, mode of mutiplication/ regeneration and quality, preferably based on active chemical constituents is also necessary this type of study, though laborious and time consuming, is nevertheless very useful. it not only provides infromation on availability of the raw material but also yields data on topographic, climatic, edaphic and hydrological condition under which the plant grows and flourishes in nature. This study also provides leads to evolve efficient methods for in-situ and ex-situ conservation as well as for domestication and cultivation. The work also includes market studies such as procurement channels of supply etc. presently, the work on these lines is limited to avery few medicinal plants raw materials. notable among these are rhizome (Sarin 1970), Rauvolfia serpentine root (Sarin 1974).

The Marketing of Medicinal Plant and Its Product in developing countries, which allow a free trade policy, is being performed in uncontrolled condition and does not possess any organised functioning pattern. The dynamism of Medicinal product Marketing largely moves around business opportunities and strength therefore, despite the competitive threats and indigenous weakness of the Medicinal Product. The status of marketing has been explained broadly as customer oriented in oligopolistics. Thus appropriate Marketing of Medicinal Product Planning for its product in term of trade channel, infrastructure, technology and behavioural dimension need to be emphasised to achieve a better economic efficiency, besides, the management consideration of Marketing – mix. It is essential to its product process in competitive scenario.

The primary level conflicts in the marketing of Medicinal products are related to the characteristics of economic environment and production. The lack of effective coordination, distribution channel, storage, packaging, branding and production process and outlets is often found to be responsible for unfavorable interactions of market forces. The marketing of Medicinal Plant objectives of the company could not be achieved for the following reasons.

(1) Mis-match of consumer demand and Medicinal product characteristics.

(2) Lack of quality and innovative concept.

(3) Absence of Medicinal Product orientation, Product line, branding and consumer awareness.

(4) In adequate communication skills and Medicinal Plant Product promotional development.

(5) Competitive, threat, higher dependency on private trade channel and lack of adequate Warehouse, Organisational arrangement for Production and Marketing of Medicinal Plants support.

It may be clearly understood that the Medicinal Plant product are competitive market oriented and cannot be sold without demand. The Product must necessarily be subject to the reasonable demand generated by existing customers as well as potential ones.

Medicinal Plant Product largely on promotional agents and distributors who push this product at a premier price and market them in high transaction places taking risk of a higher degree. The Marketing of Medicinal Products is a task which needs to perform scientifically with alternative strategies to operate in the market order to reduce dependency of Medicinal product in marketing on one channel.

Classification of Medicinal Plant

These Medicinal Products are classes into two categories viz, Manufacturer Product and consumer product.

Manufacturer product are those used for further Manufacturing processing, e.g., Medicine, cosmetic, herbal tea etc. On the other hand the consumer products mean direct use, like all food item-Amla, Hing, Pudina, Neem leaves etc.

This classification is not rigid, as some of the Manufacturer products become both consumer and manufacturer products, depending upon the use to which they are put e.g. case of dietary supplement, cosmetic, if they are consumed directly by the consumer, they become consumer product, and if the same things are used in manufacturing, they become manufacturer product.

Characteristics of Medicinal Product are divided into two categories:

(1) Production Characteristics; and

(2) Product Characteristics.

(1) Production Characteristics

(a) Small Scale Production: The production of Medicinal Plant products is carried on a very small as compared to the production of manufactured products. The techniques and principles of large scale production are not applied to a greater extent. This is particularly true in case of developing countries like India; and where 60 per cent of the total supply comes from small scale producers even in sophisticated U.S.A. and Japan, etc. In India, it is still higher. Such small production is mainly due to the small size of farms or land holdings. The Marketing of such small production creates certain problems. Marketing cannot be effective, because grading and standardisation are not possible. There is no economy in transportation. As a result, the cultivators are unable to influence the market price by individual actions. Therefore, they have to depend upon the middlemen or co-operative societies in the marketing of Medicinal Plants and its products.

(b) **Scattered and Specialised Production:** Scattered production of medicinal Plant products is a universal truth. The natural conditions like quality of the soil and climate make Medicinal production scattered and specialised. Moreover, every piece of land and every climate does not suit the production of all Medicinal Plants products. The fertility of the land varies, from place to place and particular climate and contents of the soil, and rainfall go to determine the cultivation of Medicinal Plant to be grown. As result of these peculiar characteristics of Medicinal Plants production, the process of concentration is assuming greater significance in marketing.

(c) **Seasonal Production:** Production of Medicinal Plants products are seasonal. They are not grown throughout the year. They grow only during certain months of the year, depending upon the rainfall and climatic conditions. But the demand foe them is spread throughout the year, e.g., Neem, Brahmi etc. are harvested from December to March but the demand continue. Therefore, the product move from the producing centers to the consumption centers.

(2) Product Characteristics

(a) **Variation in Quality:** The quality and quantity vary invariably from area to area. Time to time, depending on the changes in climate fertility of the soil, rainfall, art of cultivation etc. It is beyond producers to assure the quality and quantity. Because of these variation, there effects even on the storage and transport facilities.

(b) **Bulky and Perishable Products:** Medicinal Plants products are bulky in nature. The intrinsic value is quite low as compared to their bulk in appearance and size. This makes transportation and warehousing costly. Majority of the Medicinal Plant products are perishable. That is, they cannot last long. Flowers, seeds, fruits, leaves, stem, etc. are prone to perishability of high order. Therefore, they need recent improvement in refrigeration and transportation.

Recent Trend in the Marketing of Medicinal Plant Products

There have been development, even in the field of Medicinal Plant, as the there are development in research and technology, these days. The age–old traditional methods, or marketing

Medicinal Plants have been left off, and new ones have made their beginning. These recent trends can be studied under two distinct heads:

1. **Decentralisation of Marketing :** First of all, the Medicinal Plants Products used to move through channel of local market, central, Jobbing market or Secondary market and ultimately to either consumers or manufacturers. But now this trend has changed and Decentralisation has poked its nose even in the field of marketing. The central market is left aside and the Products move directly either from the producers or from the Middlemen in the local Market to the Jobbing Market or consumer or Manufacturers. These mean that there is marked change in the distribution channel and Marketing of Medicinal Plant Products is decentralised. This decentralisation is mainly due to the following factors:

(a) *Development of Modern Facility of Transportation:* Development of Modern facility of transportation has helped to cover the wide area for the collection of Medicinal Plant products. This is true, especially in case of Medicinal plants raw material like-Alovera jelly, Mint powder etc which is collected by the manufacture directly from the firms of the producers and some consumer products like-mehendi leaves etc.

(b) *The modern communication system:* The Modern communication system makes it possible to collect information about prices and supply in the market and thus, reduces the reliance on the middlemen, in the central market.

(c) *The improved warehousing facilities and cold storage arrangements:* The improved warehousing facilities and cold storage arrangements have succeeded in reducing the deterioration of quality of the products.

(d) *Standardisation grading:* Standardisation and grading, speak of quality of the products and hence the buyers donor feel like observing and inspecting the Medicinal Plant products.

(e) *The tendency of eliminating the middlemen :* The tendency of eliminating the middlemen has reached its peak, when we look at the establishment of certain large scale retail organisation like departmental stores, super market, chain stores etc of Medicinal Plant's products.

(f) *Rise and development of cooperative Marketing societies :* Last, but not the least, the rise and development of cooperative Marketing societies and regulated markets of

Medicinal Plant's Products have ensured the decentralisation process.

2. **Development of contract cultivation:** Contract cultivation of Medicinal Plants has assisted the decentralisation process. Further contract cultivation is nothing but entry into an agreement by the processors and manufacturers with cultivators to grow and supply the medicinal plants or raw material for their manufacturers. These create confidence in the producers mind and motivate them for the cultivation of Medicinal Plants products.

Channels of Distribution for the Medicinal Plants Products

The outstanding characteristics of cultivation and harvesting of Medicinal Plants have a greater and deeper bearing on the channels of distribution. The study of channels used would be most clear if tries to study, different types of Market that play constructive role in performing the function of marketing via the process of concentration, equalisation and dispersion. Because of the above reason there has been development of certain whole market which played, are playing and and will continue to play and indispensable role in the marketing of medicinal Plants. This whole markets are classed into four classes as:

1. Local Market
2. Central Market
3. Jobbing Market
4. Secondary Market

Local market: The local Market or local assembly market or growers markets or primary markets is found in the close vicinity of medicinal Plant Marketing area. It is a market where in cultivators i.e. cultivators on the one hand, consumers and intermediaries on the other, deal for the purchase and sell of firm product. They are mostly located in small town and at other convenient places. Where Medicinal Plants producer can be their produce and sell to the prospective buyers. Normally, quite a large number of whole sellers and cooperative societies operate in these markets. There main purpose is to collect or assemble the Medicinal plants products in large quantity which are to be transported later on in the central market.

1. **Characteristics of Local Market:** Absence of qualified buying- The purchase and sell are not based on the quality. The agencies in the local market do not care for quality, as

in the case showing in other market. It is because, the practices are to collect small lot of scattered production and sell without grading. Since, there is dearth or lack of specialised staffs and grading facilities and inability to cover the cost of grading, no attention is paid to quality.

2. **Careless handling:** Medicinal plant Products required lot of caution while handling them in the Marketing process e.g. leaves and stem may require good storage, packing and cold storage. Rough handling may spoil products. Therefore careful handling of Medicinal Plants Products is necessary, which is not found in the local Market.
3. **Imperfect Market:** A market is considered as perfect when there is possibility of free flow of products from one area to another area, free flow of market information via transportation and communication systems. It also calls for existence of large numbers of buyers and sellers that lead to them competition. However, due to absence of the tenets of perfect competition, we may say that there is prevalence of monopolistic market i.e. the market is less sensitive to the price changes
4. **lack of specialised services :** As compared to the terminal markets we specialised services such as grading and statanderdisation, storage etc., are conspicuous by their absence. The main reason being the agency dealing in this line is man with the little capital and with no specialised knowledge. As a result, the volume of business handled by these markets is quite small.

FUNCTION OF LOCAL MARKET

1. **Assembling of products:** the primary function of this market is to assemble the Medicinal Plants products at a single or a few points, so that they can transport economically from one point to other markets. The agency operating in this market collect the production of small lot fro individual cultivators
2. **Providing convenient place:** The local markets act as convenient place for cultivators as well as buyers. Thus, it helps the cultivators and relief them of approaching the central market and saving there time and money is also attained.
3. **Immediate cash release:** In many cases the cultivators have no patience to wait for the better prices. They want

immediate cash which is being provided by middlemen in the local market. Otherwise, the cultivators are to go to the wholesale central market and wait for the money. Thus their immediate cash requirement is availed of, by middlemen in local markets.

4. **Provision of Facilities:** Very few primary markets provide facilities of grading, storing, packing etc. But however, these are not found in all the local markets.

AGENCIES IN LOCAL MARKET OF MEDICINAL PLANTS

The following middlemen usually operate in local markets:

1. **Local resident buyers:** Local resident buyers are the persons with a fixed place of business in the local market. Their activities are limited to a single local market. They operate independently on their own or as agents of outsiders. Local residents buyers are three types:-

   (a) Retail stores.

   (b) Elevators.

   (c) Processing firms.

(a) Retail stores: Retail stores purchase mainly for selling in the local market for consumers. They are the glossary stores that buy plants parts from the cultivators and sell to the local consumers.

(b) Elevator: Elevator manufacturers refer to the merchant whose main business is to buy and sell Medicinal plants products. They buy from cultivators in the region and sell to the wholesalers in the central market. They do undertake some marketing function such as warehousing, grading and weighing etc.

(c) Processing firms : Processing firms are established either in the local market or nearer to the local market to take advantage of the assembled raw materials like – Fruits, seeds, branches, leaves etc.

(i) Traveling buyers: Traveling buyers go from one local market to another, for collecting Medicinal plants product from the cultivators. They establish their collection office at prominent places. They move from place to place in varying season. Thus they may buy the produce from growers directly or from local resident buyers.

(ii) **Cooperatives:** Cooperatives societies have been playing a note - worthy role as collecting units in the local markets.

2. **Central Market :** Central Market are also termed as terminal markets where medicinal plant's product buyers are concentrated in large volume from local markets. In this market the price locating activities operate and buyers and sellers representative the different region or nation some time meet to adjust the supply and demand of medicinal plant's product. It is the confluence of three process of marketing, viz concentration, dispersion and equalisation. The central market is located in the big thickly populated cities like-Hyderabad, Shimla, Kerala, M.P. etc. However there is no such market in the state of Jharkhand

3. **Jobbing market:** Jobbing market mainly acts as a linked between the central Market and retailers. Medicinal plant products are being bought and sold in jobbing market. The person operating are known as Jobbers These Jobbers are the whole seller operating in secondary dispersion Market. The usual products sold are – General remedies, Leaves, fruits, roots, etc. These Jobbers are intermediary who buy fro central Market, in large quantities and sell in smaller lots to the retailers.

4. **Secondary Markets :** These are also turned as sub terminal market that acts as a connecting link between the individual buyers and the central market. Secondary Market are in no way different from the Jobbing market except that the former once deal in Medicinal Plant raw material, while the later in the Medicinal plants products consumer. They supply raw materials to local manufacturers and processing firms. The medicinal raw material in which they deal are-roots, fruits, seeds, branches etc.

Channels of Distribution for Medicinal Plants Products

It is clear that the channel of distribution for Medicinal plant products is lengthier than that of the manufactured consumer products. Normally they move from producers to the resident buyers, cooperatives in the local market to the wholesale receivers, and agent middlemen in the central market to the Jobbers in the jobbing market and then to the retailers and consumers. But the channel that are in use for these consumer products, differ from producers to producers, depending on the distance between producing and consuming centers. However, the channel through which the Medicinal plant product move are:

(i) Producer-Wholesalers-Retailers-Consumers.
(ii) Producers-Retailers-Consumers.
(iii) Producer-Consumers.

(i) Producer-wholesalers-Retailers-Consumers: As we have observed earlier, the Medicinal Plant products move generally through this channel. Majority of the products are sold via this channel. In this channel, the products move from cultivator to one of the wholesalers dealing in the local market, central market and jobbing market. Thus, it is relieved by jobbers, from jobbers to retailers, who in turn sell to consumers. Since the channel is the longest one, the cost of distribution would be definitely high. Sometimes the agent middle men may also be employed. This again, adds to further cost of marketing. This is a common channel for the fresh leaves, and fruits.

(ii) Producer-Retailers-Consumers: Some Medicinal Plant consumer products such as Neem flower, leaves, and branches are being sold directly to the retailers in streets market. Thus, the producers by-pass the wholesaler in the central and local market. The retailers directly enter the local market and buy from the cultivator or producers and sell them to the consumers.

(iii) Producer-Consumer: Some medicinal consumer products are also directly by the cultivator to consumers by eliminating both wholesalers and retailers. A very small portion of the Medicinal plant products are sold through this channel. The products such as Alma fruits, karanj datum etc. are being sold directly to the consumer. Following methods are useful to sell directly :

(a) House to house selling: The products like Neem powder, Shikakai powder are sold in this way. Home delivery of the products is given. Again, the selling of Medicinal Plant's fruits and leaves by hawkers is an instance of house selling.

(b) Road side selling: The cultivator sells their products like Brahmini Leaves, Karanj Datum, Neem flowers, Amla by the side of the road, where their farm is located. This is exactly opposite of house to house selling.

(iv) Retail public market: Retail public market is the open markets where the buyers and sellers meet. The cultivator carries the goods to the particular marketplaces and sell the consumers who visit them with the purpose. In India, we call them as 'bazaars' or 'hats'. In western countries, they are commonly called as 'farmers market' or 'farmer retail market'.

(v) **Selling through post:** In advanced countries, this method is followed but this is of little importance for selling medicinal consumer products, where there is no direct touch between the consumer and cultivators, contacts are being made by means of post. According to the orders placed, products are packed and transported. It is very difficult way of selling, involves heavy cost of packing, the problem of collection and keeping of accounts.

CHANNEL OF DISTRIBUTION FOR MEDICINAL PLANTS RAW MATRIALS

The Medicinal Plants raw material passes through different channels as the consumer products do. The only difference between the two is that there are no retailers in the picture, in the channel of raw materials. The raw materials such as mint powder, satawar roots etc. are marketed through any one or more of the following channels.

1. Producer-Local Market-Central Market-Secondary market-Manufacturer user.
2. Producer-Central Market-Secondary market-Manufacturer users.
3. Producer-Secondary market-Manufacturer user.
4. Producer-Manufacturer users, directly.

The bulk of the raw material is sold through the middlemen in local market, central market or secondary market. However, direct selling is an exception.

GLARING DEFECTS OF MEDICINAL PLANTS MARKETING

The glaring drawbacks, of Indian Medicinal Plant marketing, are as many as. However, only most significant are noted here.

1. Lack of Organisation : Absence of collective organising, amongst producers, is the first defect. Unity is strength. Unfortunately, Indian farmers are widely scattered, uneducated, and freedom lovers where unit of thought, purpose and action cannot be made possible easily. However, some common union is a must to have united action in market, to protect their own interests. On the other hand, the buyers especially, the business buyers have unity. This common bargaining plays a vital role in protecting their interests.

2. Forced Village Sales: The cultivator generally sells his produce in villages, at a per cent to unfavorable place and time, and gets the lowest price. Nearly 75 per cent to 80 per cent of the output is sold in villages. It so happens because:

(a) **Indebtedness of Farmers:** Indian farmer is destined to take birth in debt, to live and to die in debt. He is in need of money for purchasing seeds, manures, and to meet expenses of the Medicinal Plant operation

(b) **Unsatisfactory conveyance System:** Even the nearest market, lacks good road system. At times, he is not having even his own bullocks or cart to move the produce to the market. Further, he does not have time to go personally to the market.

(c) **Lack of waiting capacity:** Since, many cultivation are hard pressed for cash to meet the claims of creditors i.e. money Lenders and other obligations, they are forced to dispose of the produce immediately after harvest. Thus, glut is created in the market, which results directly in the fall of prices by at least 20 to 25 per cent. Thus, the farmers get lower price.

All the above mention factors make the cultivator to sell the produce in villages only, and there by reducing there resistance power, to hold the stock of goods and reap the advantages of the market in the off season.

3. Excessive Middlemen: Indian Medicinal Plants marketing is characterised by the existence of excessive middlemen or intermediaries between the cultivator and consumer. Such a large army of middlemen which operates in the market cuts the bits both from cultivators and consumer. The cut off larger share of cake, and as a result, neither be cultivator nor are the consumers happy. It is estimated that 50 to 60 per cent of total value of communities, goes to the middlemen like wholesalers, agent middlemen, Jobbers etc.

2. Multiple Market Changes: Certain strange or peculiar practices are allowed in Indian unregulated market even today. Numerous deductions are made out of the price of produce. To get better prices the farmer carries his produce to the distant markets, where he is again cheated by the merchant. In order to dispose of the produce to the merchant. Agent middlemen, called as dealers are to be employed who charge what is known as Dalali.

3. Mal Practices in Markets: Variant mischief is being played in the market for Medicinal Plant products which are mostly unregulated. These Mal practices may be analysis follow :

(a) The producer: Seller is being goomed by buyers or middlemen in the markets by using the non standards weight and measures. To quote the experience of many villages, the middlemen use different measures and weight while buying and different measure and weight in while selling. These itself is a suffient proof of the manipulation of weights and measures by the merchants.

(b) Number of arbitrary deduction are made for religious and charitable purposes, this again reduces the share of producers – sellers in the price he gets for his products.

(c) Sufficiently large portion of produce are withdrawn as bangi or sample. Usually one – 10 seers per cartload are taken away for which nothing is paid.

(d) The brokers who are negotiating between the buyers and sellers have a tendency to favour the buyers and cheat the sellers by way of cover dealing.

(e) The buyers are in the position to dominate in case of any dispute in price, quantity, quality etc. The cultivators are not protected by any body; they are at the mercy of dealer in the market. Even it tries to protect the cultivator are-felled by shrewd business people.

(f) These and some other mal practices are experience in the unregulated Market.

4. Lack of well developed means of transportation: Transport system of our country is not satisfactory and developed even today. The development of different means of transport is very disheartening. The bad roads, and tracks which connect the villages and market, not only increase the loss of transportation, but also aggravate the strain on bullocks and other pack animals; and result is the multiplication of small dealers and intermediaries. To take the instance of construction of railways in India, the consideration which are given more weight are administrative and strategic aspects, but not the needs of the farmers. Whenever there are railway facilities, there the feeder services are not adequate and proper, as the bad roads prevent such services. The following table indicates the position of road mileage in different countries :-

Country	*Mileage*
1. France	650 miles
2. U.K	320 miles
3. USA	200 miles
4. India	100 miles

In addition to these defects, roads are not open throughout the year. Heavy rains, flood the rivers, and nalas, and the connection is cut.

5. Absence of Marketing and Standardisation: Another important defect, of our Medicinal Plant marketing system, is that the Medicinal products are not standardised and graded. The reputation, our Medicinal products, in the world market is not encouraging.

6. Lack of market Information: If at all, the cultivator is to get better prices in the market, they must know the prevailing prices. Unfortunately, cultivator has practically no contact with out side world. They depend on the hearsay reports of village's petty merchant who are least interested in supplying correct information. Even if the information is available by hard efforts, it is unrealizable because, prices are differently enforced in kilograms, tones etc. The amount of refraction differs from market to market. As a result of this, the cultivators feel to sell in villages at the price ruling there which are mostly determined by the money-lenders or village banias.

HOW TO IMPROVE THE MEDICINAL PLANT MARKETING POSITION

The discussion made until now revealed clearly, the exact mixture of the existence of defects in Marketing of Medicinal Plants products in India and the state of Jharkhand in particular. Left to themselves, the cultivators, in our country, become the scope goats of the merchant and anti-middlemen and money-lenders. If at all, the peasant in India is to obtain a higher price for his product, and the raw materials are to reach the manufacturers. In time, to carry out the cultivation of finished products, the present system of marketing should undergo through change and the whole Marketing mechanism is to be reshuffled. That is why, number of remedies is being suggested and proper steps should be taking:-

1. **Regulated markets:** Regulated market is a wholesale market where dealing or buying and selling are regulated or controlled by the state government through a "Market Committee" which consist of representatives of cultivators, traders, agents, local bodies, co-operative societies and Government. The regulated market is established with two important objectives in view viz, (a) To safeguard the interests of both cultivators and traders; and (b) To create condition of fair competition.

(a) To safeguard the interests of both cultivators and traders:-

Regulated market works under a business code of conduct framed by the "Market Committee" to be followed by cultivators and traders. Cultivators is, interested in getting higher prices for his product. On the contrary are prepared to buy more only at a low price. This may result in misunderstanding or disputes.

(b) **To create condition of fair competition:** Existence of fair competition is quite essential for the healthy growth of markets so that the fair prices can be determined. It is possible when purchase and sales are regulated by a statutory body. This is a "fair deal" in marketing the produce at an acceptable and fair price, so that the cultivator is not hit hard. The facilities of fair dealing are provided in the regulated Market.

Main Features of Typical Regulated Markets

Such a regulated market has certain characteristics of its own. They are

1. Market Committee: In accordance with the requirement of the Act a "Market Committee" is to be constituted which companies of representative from difference section of society viz., representative of cultivator, agents, traders, local bodies and co-operatives. This representative may be either elected or nominated by the government. The Market Committee enjoys certain rights and powers. It can prescribe the conditions of fair trading. Also has the right to bring about improvements in marketing methods by necessary actions and to facilitate the cultivators, at the time of marketing.

2. Methods of Sale: The Sate govt., first issues the notification in the news papers of its intention to exercise its control over trade practices in a specified area. Such an area of operation of the regulated market is laid down either as municipal limits, districts or even larger. Separate 'market yard' are necessary for effective regulation which many of the regulated market do not possess in India.

3. Methods of Sale: The main objective of regulated markets is to ensure fair trade practices, by eliminating malpractices and unauthorised deduction. In order to avoid these ills of unorganised markets, the regulated market provides for 'open auction' sale method. A representative of the market committee is to be present on the auction spot and to take note of the quantity sold, the price at which sold and the names and addresses of buyers and sellers. Thus, 'the private negotiations' are discouraged and 'underhand dealing' are prohibited.

4. Licensing the Functionaries: Those who work within the' market yard' must seek proper license from the market committee. The functionaries, who operate in the market yard, may be traders, cultivators, and other laborers. Separate license are issued to deal, in different committee. They have to procure the license after paying certain amount of fees. They have also provides the rate of commission allowances, and other charges payable to the functionaries in the regulated market.

(C) GOVERNMENT ATTITUDES TOWARDS MEDICINAL PLANTS

General

The World Health Organisation (WHO) estimated that 80 per cent of the population of developing countries rely on traditional medicines, mostly plant drugs, for their primary health care needs. Also modern pharmacopoeia still contain at least 25 per cent drugs derived from plants and many others which are synthetic analogues built on prototype compounds isolated from plants. Demand for medicinal plant is increasing in both developing and developed countries due to growing recognition of natural products, being nonnarcotic, having no side-effects, easily available at affordable prices and sometime the only source of health care available to the poor. Medicinal plant sector has traditionally occupied an important position in the socio cultural, spiritual and medicinal arena of rural and tribal lives of India.[23]

Medicinal plants as a group comprise approximately 8000 species and account for around 50 per cent of all the higher flowering plant species of India. Millions of rural households use medicinal plants in a self-help mode. Over one and half million practitioners of the Indian System of Medicine in the oral and codified streams use medicinal plants in preventive, promotive and curative applications. There are estimated to be over 7800 manufacturing units in India. In recent years, the growing demand for herbal product has led to a quantum jump in volume of plant materials traded within and across the countries. An estimates of the EXIM Bank puts the international market of medicinal plants related trade at US$60 billion per year growing at the rate of 7 per cent only. Though India has a rich bloodthirsty, the growing demand is putting a heavy strain on the existing resources.[24]

While the demand for medicinal plants is growing, some of them are increasingly being threatened in their natural habitat. For meeting the future needs cultivation of medicinal plant has to be encouraged.

According to an all India ethnobotanical survey carried out by the Ministry of Environment and Forests, Government of India, there are over 8000 species of plants being used by the people of India. Figs. 1 and 2 represents the plant in various Indian Systems of Medicine and the overlap of plant used across the medical systems.[25]

Medical Plants as Part of Culture

It is evident that the Indian people have a tremendous passion for medicinal plants and use them for a wide range of health related applications from a common cold to memory improvement and treatment of poisonous snake bites to a cure for muscular dystrophy and the enchancement of body's general immunity. In the oral traditions local communities in every ecosystem from the trans himalayas down to the coastal plains have discovered the medical uses of thousands of plants found locally in their ecosystem. India has one of the richest plant medical culture in the world. It is a culture that is of tremendous contemporary relevance because it can on one hand ensure health security to millions of people and on the other hand it can provide new and safe herbal drugs to the entire world. There are estimated to be around 25000 effective plant based formulations used in folk medicine and known to rural communities all over India and around 10000 designed formulations are available in the indigenous medical texts.[26]

Distribution of Medicinal Plants

Macro analysis of the distribution of medicinal plants show that they are distributed across diverse habitats and landscape elements. Around 70 per cent of India's medicinal plants are found in tropical areas mostly in the various forest types spread across the Western and Eastern ghats, the Vindhyas, Chottanagpur Plateau. Aravalis and Himalayas. Although less that 30 per cent of the medicinal plants are found in the temperate and alpine areas and higher altitudes they include species of high medicinal value. Macro studies show that a larger percentage of the known medicinal plant occur in the dry and most deciduous vegetation as compared to the evergreen or temperate habitats.

Analysis of habits of medicinal plants indicate that they are distributed across various habitats. One third are trees and an equal portion shrubs and the remaining one third herbs, grasses and climbers. A very small proportion of the medicinal plants are lower plants like lichens, ferns algae, etc. Majority of the medicinal plant are higher flowering plants. See Figure.

Of the 386 families and 2200 genera in which medicinal plants are recorded, the families Asteraceae. Euphorbias. Luminance,

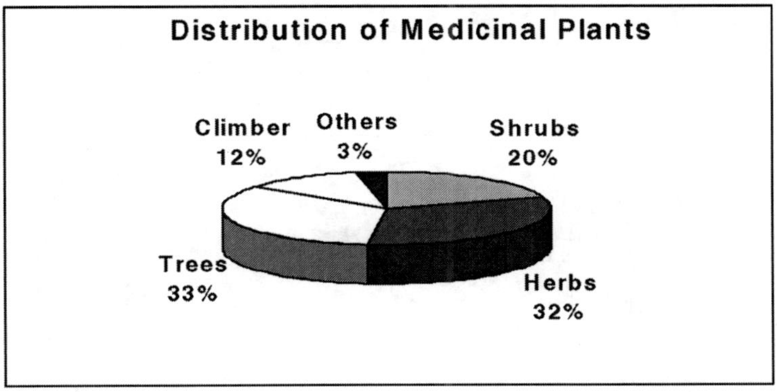

Fig. 1. Distribution of Medicinal Plants by Habits.

Fabaceous, Rubiaceae. Poaceae. Acanthaceae, Rosaceae and Apiaceae share the larger proportion of medicinal plant species with the highest number of species (419) falling under Asteraceae (See the above figure).

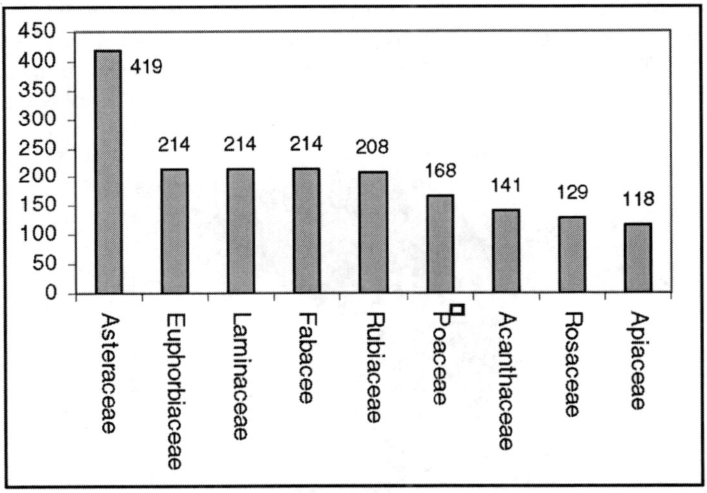

Fig. 2. Distribution of Medicinal Plant by Families.

About 90 per cent of medicinal plant used by the industries are collected from the wild. While over 800 species are used in

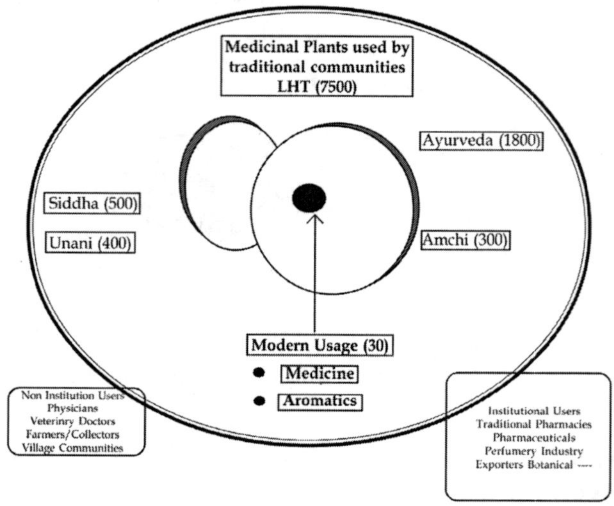

Fig. 3. Resource base of Traditional Medicine.

production by industry, less than 20 species of plants are under commercial cultivation. Over 70 per cent of the plant collections involve destructive harvesting because of the use of parts like roots, bark, wood, stem and the whole plant in case of herbs (See fig. This poses a definite threat to the genetic stocks and to the diversity of medicinal plant if bio-diversity is not sustainable used.[27]

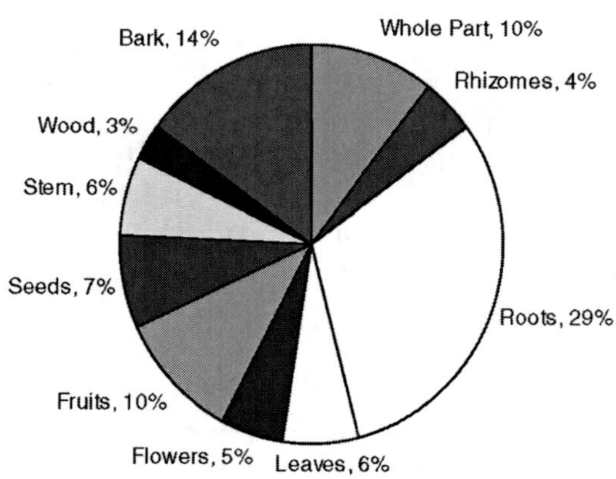

Fig. 4. Break up of Medicinal Plants by their parts utilised.

Crude Drugs and Phytochemical

Crude drugs are usually the dried parts of medicinal plants (roots, stem, wood, bark, leaves, flowers seeds, fruits, and whole plants etc.). That form the essential raw materials for the production of traditional remedies of Ayurveda, Siddha, Unani, Homeopathy, Tibetan and other systems of medicine including the fold, ethno or tribal medicines. The crude drugs are also used to obtain therapeutically active chemical constituents by specialised methods of extraction, isolation, fractionation and purification and are used as photochemical for the production of modern allopathic medicines or herbal/photoreductions. Various uses of medicinal plants are shown in the chapter.

Medicinal Plant Resource Base

Medicinal Plants are living resource, exhaustible if overused and sustainable if used with care and wisdom. At present 95 per cent collection of medicinal plant is from wild. Current practices of harvesting are unsustainable and many studies have highlighted depletion of resource base. Medicinal plants based industries although old and vast are still being managed on traditional ethos and practices and lack a proactive and sociallly responsible image. Many studies have confirmed that pharmaceutical companies are also responsible for inefficient, imperfect, informal and opportunistic marketing of medicinal plants. As a result, the raw-material supply situation is shaky, unsustainable and exploitative. There is a vast, secretive and largely unregulated trade in medicinal plants, mainly from the wild which continues to grow dramatically in the absence of serious policy attention with environmental planning. Confusion also exists in the identification of plant materials where the origin of a particular drug is a assigned to more than one plant, sometimes having vastly different morphological and taxonomical characters. There are few others, where the identify of plant sources is doubtful or still unknown, therefore, adulteration is common in such cases.

The true source of the crude drug in such cases can be located only after detailed chemical and pharmacological studies. Detailed chemical investigation on Backup monnieri and Centella Asiatic, the two plants variously described the name "Brahmi" has revealed entirely different phytochemical composition. The former contains alkaloids brahmine, herpestine, gama amino butyric acid and backside A and B which have been found to have important action on brain function, while Centella asiatica contains asiaticoside, brahmoside, hydrocotyline etc. Which have hardly common relationship with the properties ascribed to the drug "Brahmi" in the text.[28]

The quality of medicinal plants depends on the geographical origin, time and stage of growth when collection has been done and post harvest handling. The collections in most cases are done by villagers tribals residing in the vicinity of forest in their spare time. The plant part is collected without paying attention to the stage of maturity, dried haphazardly and stored for long periods under unsuitable conditions. The quality of collected material, as such is often degraded.

Trade in medicinal plants at all levels in India is marked by secrecy andopacity in working. The trade views common survey with suspicion. There has been little attempt at external regulation by Government and self-regulation by traders and herbal medicine company. However it is in the best interest of the industry to develop a long term "social contract" with the collectors or growers and buyers.[29]

Collection of Non Timber Forest Produt (NTFP), which includes most of the medicine plants, is a way of life with tribal and rural communities in an arond the forest. As the prices paid to the gatherers tend to be very low they often "mine" the natural resources as their main objective is to generate an income. A critical factor in the wild harvesting is the availability of cheap labour to undertake the very labour intensive work of gathering. As in many cases income from such sources represents the only form of paid employment for rural and tribal people, there is an eagerness to under take such work.

Several medicinal plants have been assessed as endangered, vulnerable and threatened due to over harvesting or unskillful harvesting in the wild. Habitat destruction in the form of deforestation is an added danger. The Government of India has put 29 species in the negative list of export which are believed to be threatened in the wild.

The other main source of medicinal plant is from cultivation. Cultivated material is infinitely more appropriate for use in the production of drugs. Indeed, standardisation whether for pure products, extracts or crude drugs are critical and while become increasing so, as quality requirements continue to become more stringent.[30]

Systematic cultivation of many medicinal plants needs specific culture practices and agronomical requirements. These are species-specific and are dependent on soil, water and climatic conditions.

Hence research and development work has to be done to formulate good agricultural practices which will include appropriate selection and identification, propagation methods, cultivation techniques, harvesting, step wise quality control of raw material upto processing stage, post-harvest treatment, storage and safety. These aspects have to be incorporated into protocols for the cultivation of medicinal plants.

Organic farming is another practice that is gaining wide acceptance as world demand particularly in developed countries for organically grown crops is rapidly on the increase. Farmers have to be trained in all aspects of organic farming of medicinal plants including obtaining certification from associations that do the monitoring starting from cultivation to final harvesting. Organic farming which is labour-intensive gives the developing countries the comparative advantage to be competitive.[31]

Government Attitudes towards Medicinal Plant in India

In-situ Conservation

It will be necessary, based on an understanding that where medicinal plants are currently distributed to develop novel programmes for their in-situ conservation and to designate specific genetic reserves. This intervention also applies to timber species as well as wild relative of crops, and current government activities relating to protected areas may need to be modified in order to accommodate these species. The implementation of Joint Forest Management Scheme in these areas could be a logical approach to use, given the viability of medicinal plants for generating income as well as rehabilitating degraded lands. Due to their position as the major stewards of the resource base women and tribal groups, especially, should be given some control over these lands.

The project adopted should encompass existing initiatives introduced by organisations such as FRLHT, bangalore and UTTHAN, Allahabad etc. In addition, these in-situ conservation areas should be made to serve several functions such as the provision of education and awareness building, as well as training for substantiable harvesting methods.

Ex-situ Conservation[32]

Several medicinal plants are already threatened, rare, or endangered. In addition, the "precautionary principle" applies to those where status is currently unknown and to segments of germpools. There is an immediate need to consolidate and finally link the existing herbal gardens and gene banks as well as reference specimens in herbaria to ensure that the 540 species of importance in the major classical systems, as well as those supplied to the international market, are protected in ex-situ reserves. This requires strategic planing since the range of germplasm obtained for each species must be representative. Plant collections need to evolve from being species reference collections to being genetic resources collections.

Certain plants are rich sources of intermediates used in the production of drugs. The primary processing of parts of plants containing the intermediate could be carried out in the country of origin thus retaining some value of the resource material.

Processed products (galenicals) from plants could be standardised fluid/solid extracts or powders or tinctures. Standardised extracts of many plants are widely used in health care. Some of these have to be formulated for incorporation in modern dosage forms. New formulations require some development work, particularly on account of the nature of the processed products. Plant extracts are difficult to granulate, sensitive to moisture and prone to microbial contamination. Hence the types of excipients to be used and the processing parameters have to be determined.

Quality Assurance and Standard Preparation[33]

The control of the quality of the raw materials, finished products and of processes is an absolute necessity if one is to produce goods for world market and human consumption.

International Standard Specifications exist for some processed products and some countries and buyers have their own requirements. The quality requirements for medicinal plant preparations are stringent in terms of content of active principles and toxic materials. Whereas the production of traditional medicines for local use does not require such stringent standard, what is produced will be a much more improved version of the already produced medicines using traditional methods.

Quality has to be built into the whole process beginning from the selection of propagation material to the final product reaching the consumer. It is therefore, a management system where all steps involved in the industrial utilisation process have to be properly and strictly controlled to produce the desired quality products. All elements of Total Quality Management (TQM) have to be introdeuced in any industrial project. The requirements for ISO 9000 certification and Good Manufacturing Practices (GMP) have to be introduced and the personnel trained so that enterprises could introduce the proper systems needed for certification. Furthermore eco-audit procedures (ISO 14000) leading to eco-labelling will be required for safeguarding environmental damage.

Registration and Property Rights[34]

WHO has published guidelines for the assessment of herbal medicines taking into account long and extensive usage of them (WHO, 1999). These guidelines should encourage developing countries to relax some of the current regulations to be realistic in recognising the role of traditional medicines in the health care delivery of their contries.

Attempt should be made to identify traditional health practices and knowledge relating to process and products of medicinal plants and the information should be digitised and put on computer. Where ever possible patents may be obtained for the process and products of medicinal plants.

The vital question of property right to developing countries for the use of know-how and genetic resources in the development of modern drugs has to be discussed and final solution to be derived.

Schemes of Ministry of Environment and Forests under Implementation-On-Going Schemes

National Parks and Sanctuaries[35]

The National Parks and Wildlife Sanctuaries are protected areas encompassing the Biological Diversity in its pristine condition. At present there are 87 National Parks and 447 wildlife Sanctuaries extending over an area of about 1.5 lakh sq. km, which is more than 4.5 per cent of the genographical area of the country. The National Parks stretch over 34,819 sq. km. While the Sanctuaries cover an are of 1,15,903 sq. km.

A centrally sponsored scheme for the development of National Parks and Sanctuaries is in operation since VI Plan period. The main objective of the scheme is to support protection and conservation measures in these areas with view to mitigate any adverse impact of biotic pressure and allowing the areas to rejuvenate through habitat manipulation and infrastructure development. During the VIII Plan Rs. 49.5 crores have been spent under this scheme and for IX Plan the outlay is Rs. 110 crores. Assistance is also provided for eco-development programmes around National Parks and Sanctuaries in order to achieve a ecologically sustainable economic development.

These protected areas harbor large varieties of medicinal plants. *In-Situ* conservation programmes for medicinal plants in the National Parks and Sanctuaries could be taken up through Chief Wild Life Wardens. The programme needs to be in consonance with the objectives of the national parks and Sanctuaries.

Ethnobotanically Studies[36]

An All India Coordinated Research Project of Ethnobiology (AICRPE) under the Man and Biosphere was funded by the Ministry of Environment and Forests. The programme was executed by Tropical Botanical Garden Research Institute, Thiruvananthapuram and in association with other institutions such as Central Drug Research Institute (CDRI), Lucknow, Ethnobiology and Plant Systematic Laboratory, Garhwal, Botanical Survey of India, International Institute of Ayurveda, Coimbatore, etc. The first phase of the programme was completed in 6 years and was extended into the second phase. The study has covered about 80 per cent of the tribal areas.

The Data recorded on Indian ethnobiology is invaluable giving a status on the tribal communities along with the information on the ethnobiological inventorisation and their documentation. The study provides information on the wild plants used by the tribal communities as food, fodder etc., which also includes a large number of medicinal plants.The study reveals the sustained usage of the local resoruces and the natural system of conservation. However, this natural balance is being disturbed due tothe intervention by other communities exploiting the medicinal plant resources, Data obtained from this study needs to be used in the process of planning and programme to conserve the rich biodiversity in our country. The focus on the medicinal plants resources and further investigation in these areas may lead to concrete programme for the conservation of medicinal plants.

Sacred Groves[37]

There is no separate scheme for the Conservation or restoration of sacred groves under National Afforestation and Eco-development Board (NAEB). Documentation of the Sacred Groves have been carried out by the Regional Centres of the NAEB under the scheme to “Support to Regional Centres”. There are seven regional centres and their activities include helping the State/UT Forest Departments and Forest Development Corporation in formulation of projects, conduct study research and educational programmes for the protection, development and improvement of forest area and the degraded forest areas.

Some Regional Centres have taken up the studies on the Sacred Groves under the forest protection and documentation. Such studies are proposed in the Annual Work Programme to the NAEB. The cost of the documents prepared are fixed on a case by case basis. The Work done so far included.

Sl. No.	*Sacred Grove*	*Regional Centre*	*Year*
1.	Study of sacred grove in Kurukshetra	AFC, Delhi	1996
2.	Sacred Groves of Rajastan-relevance to afforestation and eco-development	AFC, Delhi	1997
3.	Study of sacred goves in Varanasi and Mathura districts of U.P.	AFC, Delhi	N.A.
4.	Study of sacred groves of Karnataka, Kerala and Tamil Nadu	U.A.S., Bangalore	1997
5.	Sacred groves in Bihar	Jadavpur Univ., Calcutta	1996
6.	Sacred groves in Himachal Pradesh	UHF, Solan	N.A.
7.	Sacred groves of Eastern M.P.	IIFM, Bhopal	1997
8.	Sacred groves of Meghalaya	NEHU, Shilong	1995
9.	Study on the status and regeneration of forest trees in the sacred groves of Khasi Hills	NEHU, Shilong	1996

Studies have also been conducted by NGOs and research organisations to evaluate the status of sacred groves. The C.P. R. Environmental Education Centre, Chennai is one of such autonomous Centre of excellence of the Ministry of Environment and Forests. They have published books on the Sacred Trees to Tamil Nadu and Ecological Traditions of Tamil Nadu. A UNESCO study on the sacred groves of India provides a comprehensive picture of these groves along with their status. Some of the large groves and community associated with them have been presented as case studies. However, a systematic nationwide survey of sacred groves have not been undertaken to account for the status of these groves in terms of the conservation of biological diversity and the traditional particular of the community. The most important of all is the legal status and ownership of the grove. The changing pattern of life styles and religious beliefs are also responsible for the deteriorating conditions of some of the groves.

NAEB's Scheme on Non-Timber Forest Produce including[38]

Medicinal Plants

Forest areas are the main source of medicinal plants, particularly the undisturbed mutual forests. The medicinal plants from forests form an important component of the Minor Forest Produce, otherwise known as Non-Timber Forest Produce. Extraction of such produce including the medicinal plants from these areas is a traditional right of the local communicatees/tribals.

The National Afforestation and Eco-development Board (NAEB) has a mandate of promotion afforestation, tree planting, ecological restoration and ecodevelopment activities in the country. Special attention is given to the regeneration of degraded forest areas and lands adjoining forest areas, national parks, sanctuaries and other protected areas as well the ecologically fragile areas like the Western Himalayas, Arrivals, Western Ghats etc.

A Centrally Sponsored Scheme of Minor Forest Produce was started in 1988-89 (Seventh Plan). The scheme provides 100 per cent central assistance to the State and included following activities:-

(a) Mixed plantation of bamboo with fruit bearing species (harra, imli, mahua, char, aam etc. and oilseed bearing trees.

(b) Plantation of tendu bushes under light canopy of trees.

(c) Plantation of cane.

(d) Cultivation of medicinal plants like Rauwolfia spp, Dioscorea spp to augment the rising demand for plant-based drugs and to offset the scarcity because of unscientific exploitation.

(e) Cultivation of rosha grass/lemon grass.

During the Ninth Five Year Plan, the scheme is being operated in 25 States. The financial allocation is Rs. 80.50 crores. The grant released during 1997-98 and Rs. 7.50 crores and Rs. 10.00 crores respectively. The outlay for 1999-2000 is Rs. 12 crores.

The main objectives of the scheme are :

1. Conservation and improvement of the non-timber forest product, including medicinal plants;

2. Increasing the production of and replenishing the stock of non-timber forest produce and medicinal plants; and

3. Providing additional income to the tribal and the rural poor living in and around forests.

Forest Departments and Forest Development Corporation in States and Union Territories are the nodal agencies for implementation of the scheme.

Project Areas are Confined Mainly to Recorded Forest Land

JFM is a central and integral part of all plantation projects. The project authorities are being given adequate leverage by way of "entry-point activities" and requisite funds for building awareness amongst communities. In the selection of the project sites, gram panchayats or other village bodies are to be associated in project preparation, implementation and insufflate sharing in consonance with provisions of the forest (conservation) Act, 1980 and the guidelines issued in June 1990.

UNDP-CCP I assisted Sub-Programme on : "Medicinal Plants conservation and Sustainable Utilisation".

A UNDP Country Cooperation Programme assisted Sub - Programme on "Medicinal Plants Conservation and Sustainable Utilisation" has been approved and initiated in December, 1999. Foundation for Revitalisation of Local Health Traditions (FRLHT), Bangalore has been designated as the co-ordinating agency. This is a demonstration project to replicate the activities being carried out in the three Southern States of Karnataka, Kerala and Tamil Nadu and in the States of Andhra Pradesh and Maharastra. The executing agencies in Andhra Pradesh is Environmental Protection Training Research Institute (PTRI), Hyderabad and Rural Communes (RC), Mumbai in Maharashtra. The State Forest Department are the key players in the activities and would be responsible for providing the forest land for the in-situ conservation activities envisaged in the programme.

The activities include survey and inventorisation of medicinal plants in the selected areas in the State of Andhra Pradesh and Maharashtra. Identification of the sites for in-situ conservation. It would also include setting up of 8 Medicinal Plants Conservation Areas (MPCAs) in each of these states. The MPCAs thus set up would be repositories of the genetic material and the area would be demarcated as **"on harvest zones"**. One of the important features is the threat assessment of the medicinal plant species by conducting "Rapid Threat Assessment" using IUCN methodology. The programme comprises of extensive field visits and preparing herbarium sheets. The community programmes envisaged under this project would provide an opportunity for interaction and exchange of views among the different communities. Extensive training programme is also envisaged to train different section of the community, the forest officers and other field staff.

GEF Small Grants Programme

The United Nations Development Programme (UNDP) operates the Small Grant Programme on behalf of Global Environmental Facility (GEF). This provides support for small-scale community based activities which contribute to the four GEF thematic areas namely Bio-Diversity, Climate Change, Ozone layer depletion and International Waters. The SGP in India took off towards 1995 and the theme areas include Biodiversity and Climate Change. The GEF-SGP in India has been structured to operate in a decentralised manner with a National Co-ordinator based within the National Host Institution (NHI) which is Development Alternatives. A National Selection Committee (NSC) with members representing GOI, UNDP, research and voluntary organisations is responsible for overall coordination and approval of the projects.

The first phase of the GEF-SGP was set up with an initial outlay of US $ 300,000 to provide assistance to each individual project. Twenty Four projects were approved in 1995 and 1997 (20 on Biodiversity and 4 on Climate Change covering 12 States). The objectives of the programme include promoting innovative local response, capacity building, community based initiatives especially rural and tribal, create public awareness and strengthen NGOs.

The Phase-II of GEF-SGP was initiated in 1998 and the project were approved in the first meeting of the NSC held in March 1999. A sum of US $ 700,000 are made available and a number of projects on medicinal plants were considered in the meeting of NSC held. There are 11 projects on medicinal plants sanctioned under this scheme in the State of Assam, Gujarat, Himachal Pradesh, Kerala, Meghalaya, Nagaland, Rajasthan and Uttar Pradesh. These are being executed by grass root NGOs.

Future Strategies to be Adopted

For sustainable and equitable development of medicinal plant the various organisations of Ministry of Environment and Forests may adopt following strategies:

Botanical Survey of India (BSI)

The Botanical Survey of India is responsible for inventorisation of plant resources and compilation of the flora of India. The BSI may address the need for inventorisation of remaining areas. It should also update the Red Data Book of Indian Plants. It may actively focus on the ex-situ conservation of rare or threatened or endangered species of medicinal plants in various Botanical Gardens.

Indian Council of Forest Research (ICFRE)

The Institutes of ICFRE should concentrate on collection of germplasm of the 25 Plant species identified by the Task Force for cultivation. With well developed infrastructure the Institutes should try to develop agrotechnique and protocols for mass multiplication to provide quality planting material to the cultivators and foresters. It should also collect information on inter cropping rotational-cropping use of biofertilise rs and organic farming for providing know-how to the farmers and Forest Department for developing "Vanaspati Van" and cultivation of medicinal plants. The Council should attempt to make available high quality planting material by developing a network on nursery of medicinal plants. Attemps should also be made for human resource development by organising training programmes on acropathologies, post-harvest technology and quality control techniques.

Wild Life Wing of Forest Department

For conservation of medicinal plant the wild life wing of Forest Development may consider establishment of 200 Medicinal Plant Conservation Area (MPCA) covering all ecosystems, forest types and sub types in the country.

State Forest Departments

The main problems which the forest departments are facing is continuing degradation of India's forest cover, which is a source of most of medicinal plant, and it is in this extremely difficult situation that the country has to implement its commitment to the conservation of biodiversity and its sustainable use. Considering that at present 90 per cent collection of medicinal plants is from wild, generating about 40 million Mondays employment current practices of harvesting are unsustainable and responsible for depletion of resource base. To reverse this process Forest Departments have to initiate following actions.

(i) Identify forest areas rich in medicinal plants *(about 200 in number having an area of about 5000 ha)* formulate a management plan for intensive management and sustainable harvesting of herbal products.

(ii) Establishment of 200 "**Vanaspati Van**" in degraded forest areas where medicinal plants exist or existed. Each "Vanaspati Van" should have an area of **3000-5000** hectares, with irrigation facility and managed by a registered society headed by Divisional forest Officer.

(iii) It should effectively regulate extraction and transport of medicinal plants from wild. Department should maintain a list of petty traders, private agents, wholesale dealers and final consumers of medicinal plants. It should orgnise training and awareness campus on various aspects of medicinal plant development.

List of programme promotional scheme 2004-2005 project sanction by Govt. Organisation are enclosed.

Project Proposals can be Submitted in the Following Areas:

I. Promotional Schemes

1. *Survey* and Inventorisation of medicinal plants.
2. In-situ conservation and ex-situ cultivation plants.
   - To encourage in-situ conservation and ex-situ cultivation of selected medicinal plants, particularly endangered species which have appeared in Indian Red Data Book (IRDB) and negative list of CITES.
   - To create region-wise and species-wise medicinal plants demonstration centers (herbal gardens).
3. Production of quality planting material
   - To produce germ plasms of quality planting materials in bulk by developing improved agro-techniques and other appropriate technology.
4. Extension activities-Information, education and communication:
   - Awareness through audio- visual aids, talks, training, workshops etc.
   - Training and visit of growers and collectors to demonstrations plots, research centers and other related organisations in the country.

- Activities encouraging cultivation for growing medicinal plants.
- Extension material on medicinal plants.

5. Study demand supply position and marketing of medicinal plants for domestic and global market.
    - Study in respect of state-of art creating and developing infrastructure for the purpose of value addition, shelf life, storage and packing of drugs conforming international standards.
6. Research and Development in medicinal plants sector.
7. Strengthening capabilities of NMPB:- The scheme related to man-power for NMPB including pay and allowances to staff, office, infrastructure, computerisation etc.
8. Promote co-operative efforts among growers and collectors of medicinal plants.
9. Value addition and semi-processing of products of medicinal plants.
10. Undertake/assist or encourage scientific technological and economic research on medicinal plants.

Eligibility

- Applicable to government organisations for grant in the specified areas above.
- Non-Government Organisations (NGOs) and Public Sector Undertakings (PSUs) are eligible for certain specific areas except R and activities.

II. Commercial Schemes

1. Production and ensure supply of quality planting material in bulk.
2. Area expansion for selected species and cultivation in more than 2 ha. land area.
3. Value addition – for developing proper harvesting techniques, semi – processing of produces viz. collection, grading, drying, storage, packing etc.
4. Develop innovative marketing mechanism.

Eligibility

- Registered growers, association/federations of growers, traders, manufacturers, societies, pharmaceutical companies,

Public Sector Undertakings (PSUs), NGOs and recognised private research institutes or any group of people who have past 3 years experience in the medicinal plants sector.

- Government organisations.

III. Contractual Farming

Cultivation of medicinal plants on contract basis.

1. Area expansion for selected species and cultivation in commercial scale with assured market.

Eligibility

- Registered grower, association/federation of growers, traders, manufacturer, society, pharmaceutical company, NGO and recognised research institutes or any group of people who have past three years experience in medicinal plants, Public Sector Undertakings (PSUs).

Financial Assistance to Farmers

For the above commercial activies in case of ngos, societies/ cooperatives financial assistance would be provided to the extent of 30% of total expenditure, as explained above or upto a maximum Rs. 9 lacs only.

Preparation and Submission of Proposal

1. The applicant will submit the project proposal on appropriate prescribed application from **(Annexures – I, II and III)** prepared as per the guidelines of the Board. The project will have a Principal Investigator who would be responsible for its formulation and implementation.
2. The objectives of the projects have to be precise and well – defined indicating the likely benefit to be derived.
3. The technical programme of the scheme has to be as comprehensive as possible, outlining.

Exim Bank Study Highlights Export Potential of Ayurveda and Siddha Products and Services from Southern India

1. Exim Bank's latest publication titled "Exporting Indian Healthcare", highlights the prospects for export of Ayurveda and Siddha products and services from southern India and the issues involved therein. The book was released by Ms. Qudsia Gandhi, former Commissioner of Indian Medicine and Homeopathy, Government of Tamil Nadu, at a function organised by Exim Bank and CII in Chennai on October 11, 2002.

2. India has been using its rich biodiversity in the healthcare segment for many years. Its rich traditional experience and wisdom is ensconced in the Ayurveda and Siddha systems of medicine. The study explores the infrastructure facilities in the India systems of medicine highlighting the lacunae in the area of educational infrastructure, research and development, standardisation and quality control.
3. Exports of Ayurveda and Siddha products and services offer huge potential, considering that over 80 per cent of the world population relies on the traditional systems of medicines to meet their primary healthcare needs. World demend for herbal products has been growing at a rate of 10-15 per cent per annum. There is also a growing demand for natural products including items of **medicinal** value in the international **market.** The **medicinal plants** related trade in **India** alone is approximately Rs. 5.5 billion. Global market for herbal products, which include medicines, health supplements, herbal beauty and toiletry products, is estimated at around US$ 62 billion and is expected to reach US$ 16 billion by 2005.
4. The global herbal product markets. (estimated at US$ 16.7 billion in 1997) are mainly in Europe and North America, which together account for 63 per cent of the world **market.** The European **market** for herbal remedies accounts for 45% of the global **market,** and stood at US$ 7.5 billion in 1997. Germany and France are the most established markets with a **share** of 22 per cent and **11** per cent in Europe, respectively. China is the major exporter of traditional medicine to the world **market.** India needs to organise itself well to get any significant **share** in this growing **market** segment.
5. The study identifies both supply – side constraints such as lack of standardisation, lack of standardisation, lack of knowledge on international regulations governing the imports of such products, etc., as well as demand dynamics in the overseas **market,** which inhibit India's exports of Ayurveda and Siddha products and services. In addition, the issue of intellectual property is also touched upon. The challenges facing the traditional medicine system today is how to optimise the use of intellectual property by the rights holders and to prevent its abuse and misuse by non – rights holders.
6. The study concludes with a set of recommendations, at both macro and micro levels, to support the export efforts of

Ayurveda and Siddha products manufacturers and service providers in order to consolidate, mobilise and organise the sector. With global **market** growing at a much faster rate than the domestic **market,** the Ayurveda and Siddha manufacturers need to orient themselves to cater to the export needs. Organising the structure of the Ayurveda and Siddha sector and developing it as a parallel pharmaceutical industry and medical practice through modernisation and upgradation is vital for the sector to flourish.

7. Promoting Ayurveda and Siddha products and services as export items calls for as integrated effort from Government, industry, and educational and research institutions. Developing export markets would require innovative measures such as creating a few clusters – Ayurveda and Siddha cooperatives and parks. Given the support for global competitiveness by the government, possibilities of setting up Ayurveda and Siddha hospitals and centers abroad can be explored. Simultanecously, the industry needs to focus on the development of services that can be exported, and project Ayurveda and Siddha as complete health packages. The opportunities offered by exports of Ayurveda and Siddha products and services are immense and can be realised, provided persistent and focused efforts are made by all stakeholders.

References

1. Jagdish N.Sheth Bruce I.Newman, and Barbara L.Gross, "Why We Buy What We Buy" A theory of Consumption Values," *Journal of Business Research*, 22, pp. 159-70, 1991.
2. Philip Kotlar, "The Prosumer Movement: A New Challenge for Marketers," in Ritchard J. Lutz (ed), Advances in Consumer Research: Volume 13, Association for Consumer Research, Provo, UT, 1986, pp. 510-13.
3. Bernard C.Hirschman, "Primitive Aspect of Consumption in Modern American Society," *Journal of Consumer research*, 12:145, September 1985.
4. Richard N. Cardozo, "Segmenting the Industrial Market" in Robert L. King (ed), Proceeding, American Marketing Associatio, Chicago, 1968, and Richard N.Cardozo and James W. Cagley, "Experimental Study of Industrial Buying Behaviour," *Journal of marketing Research,* 8, pp. 329-334, August 1971.
5. Ajay Kohali, "Determinants of Influence in Organisational Buying : A Contigency Approach," *Journal of Marketing*, 53, pp. 50-65, July 1989.

6. Dean S. Ammer, "Top Management's view of the Purchasing Function," *Journal of Purchasing and Materials Management*, 25, pp. 16-21, Spring 1989; and Gregory D. Upah and Monroe M. Bird, "Changes in Industrial Buying : Implication for Industrial Marketers," *Industrial Marketing Management*, 9, pp. 117-21, 1980.

7. Jagdish N. Sheth, "A Model of Industrial Buyer Behaviour," *Journal of Marketing*, 37, p. 55 October, 1973.

8. Lawrence Minard, "The More it Costs the Better It Sells," *Forbes*, December 2, 1980, pp. 59-62.

9. Regis Mckenna, "Marketing in an Age of Diversity," *Harvard Business Review*, September-October 1988, pp. 88-95.

10. Sunil Mehrotra and William D. Wells, "Psychographics and Buyer Behaviour : Theory and Recent Empirical Finding," in Arch G. Woodside, Jagdish N. Seth and Peter D. Bennett (eds), Consumer and Industrial Buying Behaviour, Elsevier North-Holland, New York, 1977, pp. 49-65; and William D. Wells, "Psychographics : A Critical Review," *Journal of Marketing Research*, 12, pp. 196-213, May 1975.

11. James F. Engel, Henery Fiorillo, AN Murray A. Cayley (eds), *Market Segementation : Concepts and Applications*, Holt, New York, 1972, pp. 459-65.

12. Dennis W. Rook, "The Ritual Dimension of Consumer Behaviour," *Journal of Consumer Research*, 12 : 251, December 1985.

13. L. Bozinoff and R. Cohen, "The effects of Personal Values and Usage Situation on Product Attribute Importance, "in B.J. walker et al. (eds), An Assessment of Marketing Thought and Practice, American marketing Association, Chicago, 1982, pp. 25-29.

14. Jill Lettich, "Consumers of the '90s : Smarter and Wiser but with Less Time ," *Discount Store News*, May 7, 1990, pp. 191-92.

15. Medicinal Plant Raw materials for Indian Drug and Pharmaceutical Industry IT. Problems and prospects of Development of Resources Y.R. Sarin. The India for ester, Vol 43. 29 February 2003 No. 2 Indian medical of aromatic plants special.

16. Joshi, V.K. (2001). Market potential of plant drug used in Ayurveda. Himalayan Medicinal Plants : Potential and prospects (S.S. Samant, U.Dhar and L.M.S. Palni, eds). Gyanodya prakashan, nainital. pp. 407-414

17. Maikhuri, R.K., S. Nautiyal, K.S. Rao and K.G. Saxena (1998). "Medicinal Plant cultivation and biosphere reserve Management : A Case Study from the Nanda Devi Biospher Reserve," Himalaya. *Current Science*, 74 (2) : 157-163.

18. Maikhuri, R.K; S. Nautiyal, K.S. Rao, E.K. Chandrashekhar, R. gavali and K.G. Saxena (2000 a), Analysis and resolution of protected area-people conflicts in Nanda Devi Biosphere Reser India. Environmental Conservation, 27 (1), pp. 43-53.

19. Prasad, P.K. Chauhan, L.S. Kandari, R.K. Maikhuri, A. Purohit, R.P. Bhatt and K.S. Rao (2002). "Morchella Essulenta (Guchii) : Need for scientific intervention for its cultivation in central Himalaya," *Current Science*, 82, pp. 1098-1100.

20. Reghupathy, L. (2001). Conservation and sustainable use of Medicinal plants : current issues Himalya medicinal Plants : Potential and Prospects (S. S. Samant, U. Dhar and l. M. S. Palni, eds.). Gyanodaya Prakashan, Nainital. pp. 415-426.

21. Rao, K.S; R.K.maikhuri, S. Nautiyal and K.G. Saxena (2002). Local peoples knowledge, aptitude and perception of planning and managment issues in Nanada Devi Biosphere reserve India. Environmental Management, (in press).

22. Russel I. Haley, "Benefit Segmentation-20 Years Later," *Journal of Consumer Marketing,* 1:6 No. 2, 1984.

23. Jan- Benedict E.M Steenkamp, frenkel ter Hofstede, and Michale Wedel, "A Cross - National Investigation into the Individual and National Cultural Antecedents of Consumer Invectiveness, " *Journal of Marketing* 63, No. 7 (1999) : 55-69.

24. Melanie wallendorf, "The Formation of Aesthetic Criteria through Social Structure and Social Institution," in Jerry C. Olson, ed; Advances in Consumer Research 7 (Ann Arbor, MI: Association for Consumer research, 1980), pp. 3-6.

25. Richard T. LaPiere, Sociology, McGraw-Hill, New York, 1946.

26. Henry, "Cultural Values," pp. 121-27.

27. Michael Quinn, "Don't Aim That Pack At Us," *Time*, January 29, 1990, p. 60.

28. C.K. Prahalad and Venkatram Ramaswamy, "Co-opting Customer Competence," Harvard Business Review (January- Feb 2000):79-87. Eric von Hipple," Users as Innovators, "Technology Review 80 (Jan-Feb):3-11; Jakki Mohr, Marketing of High- technology Products and services (Upper Saddle River, NJ : Prentic Hall 2001).

29. Frank, Massy and Wind, Market Segmentation, p. 49.

30. Coleman, "The Continuing Significance," p. 274.

31. William Shakespeare, As You Like It, act 2, scene 7, lines 140-143.

32. Brad Edmondson, "How Big is the baby market?" American Demographics, December 1985, p. 27.

33. Jagdish N. Sheth Bruce I. Newman, and Barbara L. Gross, "Why We Buy What We Buy" A theory of Consumption Values," *Journal of Business Research*. 22, pp. 159-70, 1991.

34. Philip Kotlar, "The Prosumer Movement: A New Challenge for Marketers," in Ritchard J. Lutz (ed.), Advances in Consumer Research: Volume 13, Association for Consumer Research, Provo, UT, 1986, pp. 510-13.

35. Bernard C. Hirschman, "Primitive Aspect of Consumption in Modern American Society," *Journal of Consumer Research*, 12, p.145, September 1985.

36. Richard N. Cardozo, "Segmenting the Industrial Market" in Robert L. King (ed.), Proceeding, American Marketing Associatio, Chicago, 1968, and Richard N.Cardozo and James W. Cagley, "Experimental Study of Industrial Buying Behaviour," Journal of marketing Research 8: 329-334, August 1971.

37. Ajay Kohali, "Determinants of Influence in Organisational Buying : A Contigency Approach ," *Journal of Marketing*, 53:50-65, July 1989.

38. Dean S.Ammer, "Top Management's view of the Purchasing Function," *Journal of Purchasing and Materials management*, 25 : 16-21, Spring 1989; and Gregory D. Upah and Monroe M. Bird, "Changes in Industrial Buying : Implication for Industrial Marketers," *Industrial Marketing Management*, 9, pp. 117-121, 1980.

Further Reading

Jagdish N. Sheth, "A Model of Industrial Buyer Behaviour," *Journal of Marketing*, 37:55 October, 1973.

Lawrence Minard, "The More it Costs the Better It Sells," Forbes, December 2, 1980.

Regis Mckenna, "Marketing in an Age of Diversity," *Harvard Business Review*, September-October 1988.

Sunil Mehrotra and William D. Wells, "Psychographics and Buyer Behaviour : Theory and Recent Empirical Finding," in Arch G. Woodside, Jagdish N. Seth and Peter D. Bennett (eds.), Consumer and Industrial Buying Behaviour, Elsevier North-Holland, New York, 1977, pp. 49-65; and William D. Wells, "Psychographics : A Critical Review," *Journal of Marketing Research*, 12 : 196-213, May 1975.

James F. Engel, Henery Fiorillo, an Murray A. cayley (eds), Market Segementation : Concepts and Applications, Holt, New York, 1972, pp. 459-465.

Dennis W. Rook, "The Ritual Dimension of Consumer Behaviour ," Journal of Consumer Research, 12 : 251, December 1985.

L.Bozinoff and R. Cohen, "The effects of Personal Values and Usage Situation on Product Attribute Importance," in B.J. Walker et al. (eds.), An Assessment of Marketing Thought and Practice, American marketing Association, Chicago, 1982.

Jill Lettich, "Consumers of the '90s : Smarter and Wiser but with Less Time," *Discount Store News*, May 7, 1990.

Medicinal Plant Raw materials for Indian Drug and Pharmaceutical Industry IT. Problems and prospects of Development of Resources Y.R. Sarin. The India for ester, Vol 43. 29 February 2003 No. 2 *Indian Medical of Aromatic Plants Special*.

Joshi, V.K. (2001). Market potential of plant drug used in Ayurveda. Himalayan Medicinal Plants : Potential and prospects (S.S. Samant, U. Dhar and L.M.S. Palni, eds.). Gyanodya Prakashan, Nainital.

Maikhuri, R.K., S. Nautiyal, K.S. Rao and K.G. Saxena (1998). Medicinal Plant cultivation and biosphere reserve management : A case study from the nanda Devi Biospher Reserve, Himalaya. *Current Science*, 74 (2) : 157-163.

Maikhuri, R.K; S. Nautiyal, K.S. Rao, E.K. Chandrashekhar, R. Gavali and K.G. Saxena (2000 a). Analysis and resolution of protected area - people conflicts in Nanda Devi Biosphere Reserve India. *Environmental Conservation*, 27 (1) : 43-53.

Prasad, P.K. Chauhan, L.S. Kandari, R.K. Maikhuri, A. Purohit, R.P. Bhatt and K.S. Rao (2002) Morchella essulenta (Guchii) : Need for scientific intervention for its cultivation in central Himalaya. Current Science, 82.

Reghupathy, L. (2001).Conservation and sustainable use of Medicinal plants : current issues Himalaya medicinal Plants : Potential and Prospects (S. S. Samant, U. Dhar and l. M.S. Palni, eds). Gyanodaya Prakashan, Nainital.

Rao, K. S; R.K. Maikhuri, S. Nautiyal and K.G. Saxena (2002). Local peoples knowledge, aptitude and perception of planning and managment issues in Nanada Devi Biosphere reserve India. Environmental Management, (in press).

54. Nautiyal, S.K.S. Rao, R.K. Maikhuri, R. L. Semwal and K.G. Saxena (2000b). Indigenous knowledge of medicinal plants and wild edibles among three tribal sub-communities of the Central Himalyas India, *Indigenous Knowledge and Development Monitor*, 8 (2), p. 7.

Dr. D.N. Tewari, Member, Planning Commission Ex Chairman Government of India, New Delhi, No. 30015/9/99-S and T Government of India Planning Commission, Yojana Bhavan, Sansad Marg New Delhi–110 001, Dated : 14.6.1999.

Ibid., p. 4.

Ibid., p. 7.

Ibid., p. 9.

Ibid., p. 11.

Ibid., p. 14.

Ibid., p. 16.

Ibid., p. 18.

Ibid., p. 20.

Cultivation of Medicinal Plants in the state of Jharkhand, Department of Forest and Environment, published by public relation department forest advertisement and publicity, board, 2004, Ranchi, p. 8.

Ibid.

Ibid.

Ibid.

Ibid.

Ibid.

The Indian Forester, Indian Medicinal and Aromatic Plant special to volume 129, Feb. 2003, Printed by Sudhir K. Arora and Published by Neelu Gera, I.F.S, from Forest research Institute, Dehradun on behalf of the board of Management, Indian Forester. Printed at world, 29-Rajpure Road, Dehrdun. Edited by : A.K Rana, I.F.S Feb. 2003, volume 129.

4

Consumer Behaviour on Indian Environment: A General Study

Concept of Consumer Behaviour

Conceptual Approach of Consumer Behaviour and Marketing Strategic – A General Study:

The study of consumers helps firms and organisations improve their marketing strategies by understanding issues such as how

- The psychology of how consumers think, feel, reason, and select between different alternatives (e.g., brands, products);
- The psychology of how the consumer is influenced by his or her environment (e.g., culture, family, signs, media);
- The behaviour of consumers while shopping or making other marketing decisions;
- Limitations in consumer knowledge or information processing abilities influence decisions and marketing outcome;
- How consumer motivation and decision strategies differ between products that differ in their level of importance or interest that they entail for the consumer; and
- How marketers can adapt and improve their marketing campaigns and marketing strategies to more effectively reach the consumer.

Understanding these issues helps us adapt our strategies by taking the consumer into consideration. For example, by understanding that a number of different messages compete for our potential customers' attention, we learn that to be effective, advertisements must usually be repeated extensively. We also learn that consumers will sometimes be persuaded more by logical arguments, but at other times will be persuaded more by emotional or symbolic appeals. By understanding the consumer, we will be able to make a more informed decision as to which strategy to employ.

One "official" definition of consumer behaviour is "The study of individuals, groups, or organisations and the processes they use to select, secure, use, and dispose of products, services, experiences, or ideas to satisfy needs and the impacts that these processes have on the consumer and society".[1] Although it is not necessary to memorise this definition, it brings up some useful points:

- Behaviour occurs either for the individual, or in the context of a group (e.g., friends influence what kinds of clothes a person wears) or an organisation (people on the job make decisions as to which products the firm should use).
- Consumer behaviour involves the use and disposal of products as well as the study of how they are purchased. Product use is often of great interest to the marketer, because this may influence how a product is best positioned or how we can encourage increased consumption. Since many environmental problems result from product disposal (e.g., motor oil being sent into sewage systems to save the recycling fee, or garbage piling up at landfills) this is also an area of interest.
- Consumer behaviour involves services and ideas as well as tangible products.
- The impact of consumer behaviour on society is also of relevance. For example, aggressive marketing of high fat foods, or aggressive marketing of easy credit, may have serious repercussions for the national health and economy.

Applications of Consumer Behaviour

1. Marketing Strategy : The most obvious is for *marketing strategy*—i.e., for making better marketing campaigns. For example, by understanding that consumers are more receptive to food advertising when they are hungry, we learn to schedule snack advertisements late in the afternoon. By understanding that new products are usually initially adopted by a few consumers and only spread later, and then only gradually, to the rest of the population, we learn that (1) companies that introduce new products must be well financed so that they can stay afloat until their products become a commercial success and (2) it is important to please initial customers, since they will in turn influence many subsequent customers' brand choices.

2. Public Policy: In the 1980s, Accutane, a near miracle cure for acne, was introduced. Unfortunately, Accutane resulted in severe birth defects if taken by pregnant women. Although physicians were instructed to warn their female patients of this, a number still became pregnant while taking the drug. To get consumers' attention, the Federal Drug Administration (FDA) took the step of requiring that very graphic pictures of deformed babies be shown on the medicine containers.

3. Social Marketing : *Social marketing* involves getting ideas across to consumers rather than selling something.

4. Studying Consumer Behaviour: As a final benefit, studying consumer behaviour should make us better consumers.

There are several units in the market that can be analysed. Our main thrust in this research is the *consumer*. However, we will also need to analyse our own firm's strengths and weaknesses and those of *competing firms*[2]. Suppose, for example, that we make a product aimed at older consumers, a growing segment. A competing firm that targets babies, a shrinking market, is likely to consider repositioning toward our market. To assess a competing firm's potential threat, we need to examine its assets (e.g., technology, patents, market knowledge, awareness of its brands) against pressures it faces from the market. Finally, we need to assess conditions (the marketing environment). For example, although we may have developed a product that offers great appeal for consumers, a recession may cut demand dramatically.

Research Methods

There are two main categories of research methods.

1. Secondary Research uses research that has already been done by someone else. For example, marketers often find information compiled by the Indian Census very useful. However, in some cases, information specific enough to satisfy a firm's needs is not publicly available. For example, a firm will have to run its own research to find out whether consumers would prefer that more vanilla taste be added to its soft drink brand. Original research that a firm does for it is known as *primary research*.

2. Primary Research Method : There is no one perfect primary research method. Each has strengths and weaknesses, and thus the appropriate method must be selected based on research needs.

Kinds of Research

1. Survey: *Surveys* are useful for getting a great deal of specific information. Surveys can contain open-ended questions (e.g., "In which city and state were you born? ____________") Or closed-ended, where the respondent is asked to select answers from a brief list (e.g., "__Male ___ Female." Open-ended questions have the advantage that the respondent is not limited to the options listed, and that the respondent is not being influenced by seeing a list of responses. However, open-ended questions are often skipped by respondents, and coding them can be quite a challenge. In general, for surveys to yield meaningful responses, sample sizes of over 100 are usually required because precision is essential. For example, if a market share of twenty per cent would result in a loss while thirty per cent would be profitable, a confidence interval of 20-35% is too wide to be useful.

Surveys come in several different forms. Mail surveys are relatively inexpensive, but response rates are typically quite low—typically from 5-20%. Phone-surveys get somewhat higher response rates, but not many questions can be asked because many answer options have to be repeated and few people are willing to stay on the phone for more than five minutes. Mall intercepts are a convenient way to reach consumers, but respondents may be reluctant to discuss anything sensitive face-to-face with an interviewer.

Surveys, as any kind of research, are vulnerable to bias. The wording of a question can influence the outcome a great deal. For example, more people answered no to the question "Should speeches against democracy be allowed?" Than answered yes to "Should speeches against democracy be forbidden?" For face-to-face interviews, interviewer bias is a danger, too. Interviewer bias occurs when the interviewer influences the way the respondent answers. For example, unconsciously an interviewer that works for the firm manufacturing the product in question may smile a little when something good is being said about the product and frown a little when something negative is being said. The respondent may catch on and say something more positive than his or her real opinion. Finally, a response bias may occur—if only part of the sample responds to a survey, the respondents' answers may not be representative of the population.

2. Experiments : Experiments are used when the researcher wants to rule out all but one explanation for a particular observation. Suppose, for example, that we observe that sales of our brand increase when we send out coupons. However, retailers may also give us better shelf space when the coupon is out; thus, we can't tell if it was the coupon or the shelf-placement that caused sales to increase—the two variables are confounded. In an experiment, we carefully control what varies. In this case, we invite in one hundred people and ask them to shop in a simulated store. Half of the respondents are randomly selected and get a coupon; the others do not. Since the only difference here was whether the subjects got a coupon or not, we can be more confident that differences in brand choice were due to the coupon. Experiments do, however, have a serious drawback in that the consumer is removed from his or her natural surroundings. For example, if we pay some consumers to come into a lab and watch TV "as you normally would," these consumers, figuring that they are being paid, may give more attention to the advertisements than they would at home.

3. Focus Groups : Focus groups involve getting a group of 6-12 consumers together to discuss product usage. Focus groups are especially useful if we do not have specific questions to ask yet, since we don't know what consumers' concerns might be. We start out talking broadly about the need that a product might serve, and only gradually move toward the product itself. For example, a firm considering the marketing of sugar free cookies might start out its group talking about snacks—why people consume them and the benefits they expect. Gradually, we then move toward *concerns* people have about snacks. Eventually, we address sugar content and concerns that consumers have about that. Only toward the end of the session do we show consumers the actual product we are considering and ask for feedback. We postpone our consideration of the actual product toward the end because we want to be sure that we find out about the consumer's needs and desires rather than what he or she thinks about the specific product we have on the drawing board right now (that product can be changed, and it can be repositioned). Drawbacks of focus groups include high costs and the fact that generalisation toward the entire population is difficult for such small sample sizes. The fact that focus groups involve social interaction also means that participants may say what they think will make themselves look good rather than what they really believe (the social desirability bias).

4. Personal Interviews : Personal interviews involve in-depth questioning of an individual about his or her interest in or experiences with a product. The benefit here is that we can get really into depth (when the respondent says something interesting, we can ask him or her to elaborate), but this method of research is costly and can be extremely vulnerable to interviewer bias.

5. Projective Techniques: Projective techniques are used when a consumer may feel embarrassed to admit to certain opinions, feelings, or preferences. For example, many older executives may not be comfortable admitting to being intimidated by computers. It has been found that in such cases, people will tend to respond more openly about "someone else." Thus, we may ask them to explain reasons why *a friend* has not yet bought a computer, or to tell a story about a *person in a picture* who is or is not using a product. The main problem with this method is that it is difficult to analyse responses.

6. Observation of Consumers: Observation of consumers is often a powerful tool. Looking at how consumers select products may yield insights into how they make decisions and what they look for. For example, some Indian manufacturers were concerned about low sales of their products in Japan. Observing Japanese consumers, it was found that many of these Japanese consumers scrutinised packages looking for a name of a major manufacturer—the product specific-brands that are common in the India. (e.g., Hamdard) were not impressive to the Japanese, who wanted a name of a major firm like Mitsubishi or Proctor and Gamble. Observation may help us determine how much time consumers spend comparing prices, or whether nutritional labels are being consulted.

7. Physiological Measures: Physiological measures are occasionally used to examine consumer response. For example, advertisers may want to measure a consumer's level of arousal during various parts of an advertisement.

8. Segmentation : Although the text makes references to segmentation, this issue is not discussed explicitly in much detail. However, segmentation is important in consumer analysis because understanding the consumer will allow us segment the market more meaningfully.

Segmentation basically involves dividing consumers into groups such that members of a group (1) are as similar as possible to members of that same group but (2) differ as much as possible from members other segments. This enables us then to "treat" each segment differently—e.g., by:

- Providing different products (e.g., some consumers like Zandu taste, while others prefer Dabur)

- Offering different prices (some consumers will take the cheapest product available, while others will pay for desired features)
- Distributing the products where they are likely to be bought by the targeted segment.

In order for a segment structure to be useful:

- Each segment must have an identity—i.e., it must contain members that can be described in some way (e.g., price sensitive) that behave differently from another segment.
- Each segment must engage in systematic behaviours (e.g., a price sensitive segment should consistently prefer the low price item rather than randomly switching between high and low priced brands).
- Each segment must offer marketing mix efficiency potential—i.e., it must be profitable to serve. For example, a large segment may be profitable even though the competition it attracts tends to keep prices down. A smaller segment may be profitable if, for example, it is price insensitive or can be targeted efficiently (e.g., if its members consistently subscribe to one magazine where all the company's advertising can be put). Some segments are not cost effective. For example, a small group of consumers would love to have a no-sports news channel (similar to NDTV), but we are just too small a group to profitable.

There are three "levels" of segmentation. Levels here refer to the trade-off between the difficulty of implementing a segmentation scheme and the benefits that result.[3]

1. Personal Characteristics : The first level of segmentation involves *personal characteristics*—e.g., demographics. This is a fairly easy method of segmentation to employ because (1) we have a good idea of who is in each segment and (2) we can easily target these segments. For example, if we want to reach males ages fifteen through thirty-five, we can find out which TV shows they watch from firms. The trouble with this method of segmentation, however, is that there is often not a good correlation between personal characteristics of consumers and what they want to buy. Perhaps males may want more flavor, and be willing to settle for more calories, in a soft drink than women do, but there is a great deal of within group variation. Interestingly, it has been found that people who live in the same area, as operational sed by their zip codes, tend to share a many consumption relevant characteristics. Firms such as Dabur/Zandu will sell profiles of zip code based communities that can be used in aiming messages at particularly receptive residents.

Psychographies includes a bit more information about the consumer than his or her mere descriptive characteristics. For example, two men could both be plumbers, aged 45, married with two children, and have annual incomes of 45,000. However, one could be couch potato who comes home and eats fast food while watching television. The other could be a health enthusiast who spends his time exercising. Several firms have tried to come up with psychographic profiles of consumers.[4]

2. The Second Level is Benefit Desired: That is, segmenting on what someone wants rather than who he or she is. Implementing segmentation on benefit desired is more difficult since we have to research for each product category. The benefit, however, is that we can now make product that matches more closely a particular segment's specific desires, and we can promote, price, and distribute it according to the desires of the segment. This method, then, lends itself extremely well to strong product positioning—we make a product that offers specific benefits, and we aggressively promote this fact to interested consumers. A drawback, however, is some efficiency is lost in marketing communication. While we can look up which television programs males ages twenty to thirty watch, we do not have this information for the segment of consumers that prefers scented over unscented hand soap.

3. The Third Level is Segmentation Based on Behaviour: Behaviour here refers to a person's response (or lack of response) to a given treatment. For example, some consumers will switch from their preferred brand to another one that happens to be on sale (the "switchers,") while others will stay with the preferred brand (the "loyal.") The trick, then, is to get as many switchers as possible to switch to your brand (which will take some incentive, such as a cents off coupon) while not giving this incentive to the brand loyal (who would have bought your brand even without the discount). In practice, segmenting on behaviour can be very difficult. For example, supermarkets spend a great deal of money to establish the "clubs" that give price sensitive customers who are willing to go through with the required paperwork discounts not available to the "lazier" ones that end up paying full price. Despite this difficulty, the rewards are often great; because we can tailor the kind of deal we give a consumer to the minimum concession needed to get that consumer to buy our (as opposed to a competing) product.

Direct Marketing Offers exceptional opportunities for segmentation because marketers can buy lists of consumer names, addresses, and phone-numbers that indicate their specific interests. For example, if we want to target auto enthusiasts, we can buy lists of subscribers to auto magazines and people who have bought auto supplies through the mail. We can also buy lists of people who have particular auto makes registered.

No One List will Contain all the Consumers we want, and in recent years technology has made it possible, through the "*merge-purge*" process, to combine lists. For example, to reach the above-mentioned auto-enthusiasts, we buy lists of subscribers to several different car magazines, lists of buyers from the Hot Wheels and Wiring catalog, and registrations of Porsche automobiles in several states. We then combine these lists (the *merge* part). However, there will obviously be some overlap between the different lists—some people subscribe to more than one magazine, for example. The *purge* process, in turn, identifies and takes out as many duplicates as possible. This is not as simple task as it may sound up front. For example, the address "123 Main Street, Apartment 45" can be written several ways—e.g., 123 Main St., #123, or 123-45 Main Str. Similarly, Ravi. Vijay. Verma could also be written as R. V. Verma, (e.g., all street addresses would be converted into the format "123 Main St #45" and even uses phonetic analysis to identify a likely alternative spelling of the same name.[5]

Response Rates for "Good" lists—lists that represent a logical reason why consumer would be interested in a product—are typically quite low, hovering around 2-3%. Simply picking a consumer out of the phone book would yield even lower responses—much less than one per cent. Keep in mind that a relevant comparison here is to conventional advertising. The response rate to an ad placed in the newspaper or on television is usually well below one per cent (frequently more like one-tenth of one per cent). (More than one per cent of people who see an ad for Coke on TV will buy the product, but most of these people would have bought Coca Cola anyway, so the *marginal* response is low).

Philosophy of Culture

Culture is part of the *external* influences that impact the consumer. That is, culture represents influences that are imposed on the consumer by other individuals.

The definition of culture offered in the text is "That complex whole which includes knowledge, belief, art, morals, custom, and any other capabilities and habits acquired by man person as a member of society". From this definition, we make the following observations:[6]

- Culture, as a "complex whole," is a system of interdependent components.
- Knowledge and beliefs are important parts. In India, we know and believe that a person who is skilled and works hard will get ahead. In other countries, it may be believed that differences in outcome result more from luck. "Chinking," the name for China in Chinese, literally means "The Middle Kingdom." The belief among ancient Chinese that they were in the center of the universe greatly influenced their thinking.
- Other issues are relevant. Art, for example, may be reflected in the rather arbitrary practice of wearing ties in some countries and wearing turbans in others. Morality may be exhibited in the view in India that one should not be naked in public. In Japan, on the other hand, groups of men and women may take steam baths together without perceived as improper. On the other extreme, women in some Arab countries are not even allowed to reveal their faces. Notice, by the way, that what at least some countries view as moral may in fact be highly immoral by the standards of another country.
- Culture has several important characteristics: (1) Culture is *comprehensive*. This means that all parts must fit together in some logical fashion. For example, bowing and a strong desire to avoid the loss of face are unified in their manifestation of the importance of respect. (2) Culture is *learned* rather than being something we are born with. We will consider the mechanics of learning later in the course. (3) Culture is manifested within *boundaries* of acceptable behaviour. (4) Conscious awareness of cultural standards is limited. (5) Cultures fall somewhere on a continuum between static and dynamic depending on how quickly they accept change. For example, American culture has changed a great deal since the 1950s, while the culture of India has changed much less.

It should be noted that there is a tendency of outsiders to a culture to overstate the similarity of members of that culture to each other between social classes.

Cultural rules can be categorised into three types. *Formal rules* carry relatively explicit standards as to how one should behave, and violations often carry severe sanctions. For example, in many countries, two forms of the second pronoun (you) exist, with different levels of deference associated with each (In Japan, senior executives will enter and leave a meeting room before subordinates in a very deliberate manner. *Informal rules*, on the other hand, are less explicit and may not carry sanctions for violation. Language is an important element of culture. It should be realised that regional differences might be subtle. For example, one word may mean one thing, but something off-color in another. It should also be kept in mind that much information is carried in non-verbal communication. In some cultures, we nod to signify "yes" and shake our heads to signify "no;" in other cultures, the practice is reversed.[7]

Different perspectives exist in different cultures on several issues; e.g.:

- *Monochromic* cultures tend to value precise scheduling and doing one thing at a time; in *polyphonic* cultures, in contrast, promptness is valued less, and multiple tasks may be performed simultaneously.
- *Space* is perceived differently. India will feel crowded where people from more densely populated countries will be comfortable.
- In the U.S. and much of Europe, agreements are typically rather precise and contractual in nature; in Asia, there is a greater tendency to settle issues as they come up. As a result, building a relationship of trust is more important in Asia, since you must be able to count on your partner being reasonable.
- In terms of etiquette, some cultures have more rigid procedures than others. In some countries, for example, there are explicit standards as to how a gift should be presented. In some cultures, gifts should be presented in private to avoid embarrassing the recipient; in others, the gift should be made publicly to ensure that no perception of secret bribery could be made.

Culture in Indian Context

The Indian has undergone some changes in its predominant culture over the last several decades. Again, however, it should be kept in mind that there are great variations within the culture. For example, on the average, Indian has become less materialistic and has sought more leisure; on the other hand, the percentage of people working extremely long hours has also increased. The text discusses changes in values in more detail.[7]

Significant changes have occurred in gender roles in Indian society. One of the reasons for this is that more women work outside the home than before. However, women still perform a disproportionate amount of housework, and men who participate in this activity tend to do so reluctantly. In general, commercials tend to lag somewhat behind reality—e.g., few men are seen doing housework, and few women are seen as buyers and decision makers on automobile purchases.

Subculture refers to a culture within a culture. For example, Indian are as indicated in the group name, Indian For example, although this does not apply to everyone, Indian tend to worship in Holy places that have predominantly, Different perspectives on the diversity in Indian culture exist. The "melting pot" metaphor suggests that immigrants gradually assimilate after they arrive. Therefore, in the long run, there will be few differences between ethnic groups and instead, one mainstream culture that incorporates elements from each will result. The "salad bowl" metaphor, in contrast, suggests that although ethnic groups will interact as a whole (through the whole mix of salad) and contain some elements of the whole (through the dressing), each group will maintain its own significant traits (each vegetable is different from the others). The "melting pot" view suggests that one should run integrated promotions aimed at all groups; the "salad bowl" approach suggests that each group should be approached separately.[8]

Subculture is often categorised on the basis of demographics. Values are often greatly associated with age groups because people within an age group have shared experiences. For example, it is believed that people old enough to have experienced the Indian Depression are more frugal because of that experience.

Demographics and Social Stratification

Demographics are clearly tied to subculture and segmentation. Here, however, we shift our focus from analysing specific subcultures to trying to understand the implications for an entire population of its makeup.

Several issues are useful in the structure of a population. For example, in some rapidly growing countries, a large percentage of the population is concentrated among younger generations. In countries such as Korea, China, and Taiwan, this has helped stimulate economic growth, while in certain poorer countries; it puts pressures on society to accommodate an increasing number of people on a fixed amount of land.

Family Decision Making

The Family Life Cycle. Individuals and families tend to go through a "life cycle." The simple life cycle goes from

Child/teenager → young single → young couple* → full nest → Empty nest → widow.

In real life, this situation is, of course, a bit more complicated. For example, many couples undergo divorce. Then we have the scenario:

Full nest → single parent

This situation can result either from divorce or from the death of one parent. Divorce usually entails a significant change in the relative wealth of spouses. In some cases, the noncustodial parent (usually the father) will not pay the required child support, and even if he or she does, that still may not leave the custodial parent and children as well off as they were during the marriage. On the other hand, in some cases, some noncustodial parents will be called on to pay a large part of their income in child support. This is particularly a problem when the noncustodial parent remarries and has additional children in the second (or subsequent marriages). In any event, divorce often results in a large demand for:

- Low cost furniture and household items
- Time-saving goods and services

Divorced parents frequently remarry, or become involved in other non-marital relationships; thus, we may see

Full nest → single parent → blended family

Another Variation Involves

Young single → single parent

Here, the single parent who assumes responsibility for one or more children may not form a relationship with the other parent of the child.

Generally, there are two main themes in the Family Life Cycle, subject to significant exceptions:[9]

*For purposes of this discussion, a "couple" may either be married or merely involve living together. The breakup of a non-marital relationship involving cohabitation is similarly considered equivalent to a divorce.

1. As a person gets older, he or she tends to advance in his or her career and tends to get greater income (exceptions: maternity leave, divorce, retirement).
2. Unfortunately, obligations also tend to increase with time (at least until one's mortgage has been paid off). Children and paying for one's house are two of the greatest expenses.

Note that although a single person may have a lower income than a married couple, the single may be able to buy more discretionary items.

Family Decision Making: Individual members of families often serve different roles in decisions that ultimately draw on shared family resources. Some individuals are *information gatherers/ holders*, who seek out information about products of relevance. These individuals often have a great deal of power because they may selectively pass on information that favors their chosen alternatives. *Influencer* do not ultimately have the power decide between alternatives, but they may make their wishes known by asking for specific products or causing embarrassing situations if their demands are not met. The *decision maker(s)* have the power to determine issues such as:

- Whether to buy;
- Which product to buy (pick-up or passenger car?);
- Which brand to buy;
- Where to buy it; and
- When to buy.

Note, however, that the role of the decision maker is separate from that of the *purchaser*. From the point of view of the marketer, this introduces some problems since the purchaser can be targeted by point-of-purchase (POP) marketing efforts that cannot be aimed at the decision maker. Also note that the distinction between the purchaser and decision maker may be somewhat blurred:

- the decision maker may specify what kind of product to buy, but not which brand;
- the purchaser may have to make a substitution if the desired brand is not in stock;
- the purchaser may disregard instructions (by error or deliberately).

It should be noted that family decisions are often subject to a great deal of conflict. The reality is that few families are wealthy enough to avoid a strong tension between demands on the family's resources. Conflicting pressures are especially likely in families with children and/or when only one spouse works outside the home. Note that many decisions inherently come down to values, and that there is frequently no "objective" way to arbitrate differences. One spouse may believe that it is important to save for the children's future; the other may value spending now (on private schools and computer equipment) to help prepare the children for the future. Who is right? There is no clear answer here. The situation becomes even more complex when more parties—such as children or other relatives—are involved.

Some family members may resort to various strategies to get their way. One is *bargaining*—one member will give up something in return for someone else. For example, the wife says that her husband can take an expensive course in gourmet cooking if she can buy a new pickup truck. Alternatively, a child may promise to walk it every day if he or she can have a hippopotamus. Another strategy is *reasoning*—trying to get the other person(s) to accept one's view through logical argumentation. Note that even when this is done with a sincere intent, its potential is limited by legitimate differences in values illustrated above. Also note that individuals may simply try to "wear down" the other party by endless talking in the guise of reasoning (this is a case of *negative reinforcement* as we will see subsequently). Various manipulative strategies may also be used. One is *impression management*, where one tries to make one's side look good (e.g., argue that a new TV will help the children see educational TV when it is really mostly wanted to see sports programming. *Authority* involves asserting one's "right" to make a decision (as the "man of the house," the mother of the children, or the one who makes the most money). *Emotion* involves making an emotional display to get one's way.

Group Influences

Humans are inherently social animals, and individuals greatly influence each other.[10]

A useful framework of analysis of group influence on the individual is the so-called *reference group*—the term comes about because an individual uses a relevant group as a standard of reference against which oneself is compared. Reference groups come in several different forms. The *inspirational reference group* refers to those others against whom one would like to compare oneself. For example, many firms use athletes as spokes people, and these represent what many people would ideally like to be.

Associative reference groups include people who more realistically represent the individuals' current equals or near-equals—e.g. neighbours, clubs, and organisations. Finally, the *dissociate* reference group includes people that the individual would *not* like to be like. For example, the store literally named The Gap came about because many younger people wanted to actively dissociate from parents and other older and "uncool" people. The Quality Paperback Book specifically suggests in its advertising that its members are "a breed apart" from conventional readers of popular books.

Reference groups come with various degrees of influence. *Primary* reference groups come with a great deal of influence—e.g., members of a fraternity/sorority. *Secondary* reference groups tend to have somewhat less influence—e.g., members of a boating club that one encounters only during week-ends are likely to have their influence limited to consumption during that time period.

Another typology divides reference groups into the *informational* kind (influence is based almost entirely on members' knowledge), *normative* (members influence what is perceived to be "right," "proper," "responsible," or "cool"), or *identification*. The difference between the latter two categories involves the individual's motivation for compliance. In case of the normative reference group, the individual tends to comply largely for utilitarian reasons—dressing according to company standards is likely to help your career, but there is no real motivation to dress that way outside the job. In contrast, people comply with identification groups' standards for the sake of belonging—for example, a member of a religious group may wear a symbol even outside the house of worship because the religion is a part of the person's identity.

Diffusion of Innovation

The diffusion of innovation refers to the tendency of new products, practices, or ideas to spread among people. Usually, when new products or ideas come about, they are only adopted by a small group of people initially; later, many innovations spread to other people. The bell shaped curve frequently illustrates the rate of adoption of a new product. Cumulative adoptions are reflected by the S-shaped curve. The *saturation point* is the maximum proportion of consumers likely to adopt a product.[11]

Several specific product categories have case histories that illustrate important issues in adoption. Until some time in the 1800s, few physicians bothered to scrub prior to surgery, even though new scientific theories predicted that small microbes not visible to the naked eye could cause infection. Younger and more progressive physicians began scrubbing early on, but they lacked the stature to make their older colleagues follow.

ATM cards spread relatively quickly. Since the cards were used in public, others who did not yet hold the cards could see how convenient they were. Although some people were concerned about security, the convenience factors seemed to be a decisive factor in the "tug-of-war" for and against adoption.

The case of credit cards was a bit more complicated and involved a "chicken-and-egg" paradox. Accepting credit cards was not a particularly attractive option for retailers until they were carried by a large enough number of consumers. Consumers, in contrast, were not particularly interested in cards that were not accepted by a large number of retailers. Thus, it was necessary to "jump start" the process, signing up large corporate accounts, under favorable terms, early in the cycle, after which the cards became worthwhile for retailers to accept.

Remix music initially spread quickly among urban youths in large part because of the low costs of recording. Later, remix music became popular among a very different segment, suburban youths, because of its apparently authentic depiction of an exotic urban life-style.

Hybrid seeds were adopted only slowly among many farmers. Although hybrid seed provided yields of about 40 per cent more than traditional seed, many farmers had difficulty believing that this smaller seed could provide a superior harvest. They were usually reluctant to try it because a failed harvest could have serious economic consequences, including a possible loss of the farm. Agricultural extension agents then sought out the most progressive farmers to try hybrid seeds, also aiming for farmers who were most respected and most likely to be imitated by others. Few farmers switched to hybrid seed outright from year to year. Instead, many started out with a fraction of their land, and gradually switched to 100 per cent hybrid seed when this innovation had proven itself useful.

Several forces often work against innovation. One is risk, which can be either social or financial. For example, early buyers of the CD player risked that few CDs would be recorded before the CD player went the way of the 8 track player. Another risk is being perceived by others as being weird for trying a "fringe" product or idea. Compatibility with the existing culture or technology. For example, birth control is incompatible with strong religious influences in countries heavily influenced by Hindu/Islam or Catholicism/Sikh.

Innovations come in different degrees. A *continuous* innovation includes slight improvements over time. Very little usually changes from year to year in automobiles, and even automobiles of the 1990s are driven much the same way that automobiles of the 1950 were driven. A *dynamically continuous* innovation involves some change in technology, although the product is used much the same way that its predecessors were used—e.g., jet vs. Propeller aircraft. A *discontinuous* innovation involves a product that fundamentally changes the way that things are done—e.g., the fax and photocopiers. In general, discontinuous innovations are more difficult to market since greater changes are required in the way things are done, but the rewards are also often significant.

Several factors influence the speed with which an innovation spreads. One issue is relative advantage (i.e., the ratio of risk or cost to benefits). Some products, such as cellular phones, fax machines, and ATM cards, have a strong relative advantage. Other products, such as automobile satellite navigation systems, entail some advantages, but the cost ratio is high. Lower priced products often spread more quickly, and the extent to which the product is *trial able* (farmers did not have to plant all their land with hybrid seed at once, while one usually has to buy a cellular phone to try it out) influence the speed of diffusion. Finally, the extent of switching difficulties influences speed—many offices were slow to adopt computers because users had to learn how to use them.

Some cultures tend to adopt new products more quickly than others, based on several factors:

- *Modernity*: The extent to which the culture is receptive to new things
- *Homophile:* The more similar to each other that members of a culture are, the more likely an innovation is to spread—people are more likely to imitate similar than different models. *Physical distance:* The greater the distance between people, the less likely innovation is to spread.
- *Opinion leadership:* The more opinion leaders are valued and respected, the more likely and innovation is to spread. The style of opinion leaders moderates this influence, however. In less innovative countries, opinion leaders tend to be more conservative, i.e., to reflect the local norms of resistance.

It should be noted that innovation is not always an unqualifiedly good thing. Some innovations, such as infant formula adopted in developing countries, may do more harm than good. Individuals may also become dependent on the innovations. For example, travel agents who get used to booking online may be unable to process manual reservations.

Sometimes innovations are disadopted. For example, many individuals disadopt cellular phones if they find out that they don't end up using them much.

Perception

Background: Our perception is an approximation of reality. Our brain attempts to make sense out of the stimuli to which we are exposed. This works well, for example, when we "see" a friend three hundred feet away at his or her correct height; however, our perception is sometimes "off"—for example, certain shapes of ice cream containers look like they contain more than rectangular ones with the same volume.[12]

Factors in perception: Several sequential factors influence our perception. *Exposure* involves the extent to which we encounter a stimulus. For example, we are exposed to numerous commercial messages while driving on the freeway: bill boards, radio advertisements, bumper-stickers on cars, and signs and banners placed at shopping malls that we pass. Most of this exposure is random—we don't plan to seek it out. However, if we are shopping for a car, we may deliberately seek out advertisements and "tune in" when company advertisements come on the radio/TV.

Exposure is not enough to significantly impact the individual—at least not based on a single trial (certain advertisements, or commercial exposures)). In order for stimuli to be consciously processed, *attention* is needed. Attention is actually a matter of degree—our attention may be quite high when we read directions for getting an income tax refund, but low when commercials come on during a television programme. Note, however, that even when attention is low, it may be instantly escalated—for example, if an advertisement for a product in which we are interested comes on.

Interpretation involves making sense out of the stimulus. For example, when we see a red can, we may categorise it as a Coke.

Several factors influence the extent to which stimuli will be noticed. One obvious issue is *relevance*. Consumers, when they have a choice, are also more likely to attend to *pleasant* stimuli (but when the consumer can't escape, very unpleasant stimuli are also likely to get attention—thus, many very irritating advertisements are remarkably effective).

Surprising stimuli are likely to get more attention—survival instinct requires us to give more attention to something unknown that may require action. A greater *contrast* (difference between the stimulus and its surroundings) as well as greater *prominence* (e.g., greater size, center placement) also tends to increase likelihood of processing.

Learning and Memory

Background. Learning involves "a change in the content or organisation of long term memory and/or behaviour." The first part of the definition focuses on what we know (and can thus put to use) while the second focuses on concrete behaviour. For example, many people will avoid foods that they consumed shortly before becoming ill. Learning is not all knowledge based. For example, we may experience the sales people in one store being nicer to us than those in the other. We thus may develop a preference for the one store over the other; however, if pressed, we may not be able to give a conscious explanation as to the reason for our preference.[13]

Much early work on learning was actually done on rats and other animals (and much of this research was unjustifiably cruel, but that is another matter).

Operant conditioning. Instrumental, or operant, conditioning, involves a different series of events, and this what we usually think of as learning. The general pattern is:

Behaviour → consequences → behaviour is more or less likely to be repeated

There are three major forms of operant learning. In *positive reinforcement*, an individual does something and is rewarded. He or she is then more likely to repeat the behaviour. For example, you eat a candy bar (behaviour), it tastes good (consequence), and you are thus more likely to eat a similar candy bar in the future (behavioural change).

Punishment is the opposite. You eat what looks like a piece of candy (behaviour), only to discover that it is a piece of soap with a foul taste (consequences), and subsequently you are less likely to eat anything that looks remotely like that thing ever again (changed behaviour).

It should be noted that *negative reinforcement* is very different from punishment. An example of negative reinforcement is an obnoxious sales person who calls you up on the phone, pressuring you into buying something you don't want to do (aversive stimulus). You eventually agree to buy it (changed behaviour), and the sales person leaves you alone (the aversive stimulus is terminated as a result of consequences of your behaviour).

In general, marketers usually have relatively little power to use punishment or negative reinforcement.

Several factors influence the effectiveness of operant learning. In general, the *closer in time* the consequences are to the behaviour, the more effective the learning. That is, electric utilities would be more likely to influence consumers to use less electricity at peak hours if the consumers actually had to pay when they used electricity rather than at the end of the month. Learning is also more likely to occur when the individual can *understand a relationship* between behaviour and consequences (but learning may occur even if this relationship is not understood consciously).

Another issue is schedules of reinforcement and *extinction*. Extinction occurs when behaviour stops having consequences and the behaviour then eventually stops occurring. For example, if a passenger learns that yelling at check-in personnel no longer gets her upgraded to first class, she will probably stop that behaviour. Sometimes, an individual is rewarded every time a behaviour is performed (e.g., a consumer gets a Weight card every time coins are put into a weigh machine). However, it is not necessary to reward a behaviour every time for learning to occur. Even if a behaviour is only rewarded some of the time, the behaviour may be learned. Several different *schedules of reinforcement* are possible:[14]

- *Fixed interval*: The consumer is given a free dessert on every Sunday when he or she eats in a particular restaurant.
- *Fixed ratio*: Behaviour is rewarded (or punished) on every *n*th occasion that it is performed. (e.g., every tenth time a frequent shopper card is presented, a free product is provided).
- *Variable ratio*: Every time an action is performed, there is a certain percentage chance that a reward will be given. For example, every time the consumer enters the store, he or she is given a lottery ticket. With each ticket, there is a 20% chance of getting a free T-Shirt. The consumer may get a free T-Shirt twice in a row, or he or she may go ten times without getting a T-Shirt even once.

Variable Ratio Reinforcement is Least Vulnerable to Extinction

Sometimes, *shaping* may be necessary to teach the consumer the desired behaviour. That is, it may be impossible to teach the consumer to directly perform the desired behaviour. For example, a consumer may first get a good product for free (the product itself, if good, is a reward), then buy it with large cents off coupon, and finally buy it at full price. Thus, we reinforce approximations of the desired behaviour.

Vicarious learning. The consumer does not always need to go through the learning process himself or herself—sometimes it is possible to learn from observing the consequences of others. For example, stores may make a big deal out of prosecuting shoplifters not so much because they want to stop that behaviour in the those caught, but rather to deter the behaviour in others. Similarly, viewers may empathise with characters in advertisements that experience (usually positive) results from using a product. The Head 'n' Shoulders advertisement, where a poor man is rejected by women until he treats his dandruff with an effective cure, is a good example of *vicarious learning.*

Memory. There are two kinds of memory. When you see an ad on TV for a mail order product you might like to buy, you only keep the phone number in memory until you have dialed it. This is known as *short-term* memory. In order for something to enter into *long-term* memory, which is more permanent, you must usually "rehearse" it several times. For example, when you move and get a new phone number, you will probably repeat it to yourself many times. Alternatively, you get to learn your driver's license or social security numbers with time, not because you deliberately memorise them, but instead because you encounter them numerous times as you look them up.

A special issue in memory is so called "scripts," or procedures we remember for doing things. Scripts involve a series of steps for doing various things (e.g., how to send a package). In general, it is useful for firms to have their brand names incorporated into scripts (e.g., to have the consumer reflexively ask the pharmacist for Buyer rather than an unspecified brand of aspirin).

Motivation, Personality and Emotion

Perspectives on Consumer Behaviour and Motivation. We considered several perspectives on behaviour as a way to understand what motivates the consumer. Each of these perspectives suggests different things as to what the marketer should do and what can (and cannot) be controlled. Note that each perspective tends to contain a "grain" of truth and that one should not be too dogmatic in emphasising one over the others.[15]

- **The *Hard Core Behavioural* perspective** is based on learning theories such as operant and classical conditioning. These theories suggest that consumers must learn from their own experiences—i.e. in order to avoid getting sick from overeating, a consumer must experience the stomach and other ailments resulting from gluttony rather than merely observing *other people* who overeat and get sick. This suggests, then, that it is important to reward good behaviour (e.g., buying our brand) to the extent possible. Money spent on advertising is seen as less useful. Hard core behaviourists tend to look at observable behaviour (e.g., buying our brand *or* buying another) rather than trying to find out what is going on inside the heads of consumers—i.e., hard core behaviourists do not like to mess with "mushy" things like attitudes.
- **The *Social Learning Perspective*,** in contrast, allows for *vicarious* learning—i.e. learning obtained by watching others getting good or bad consequences for behaviour. The *models* that may be observed and imitated include peers and family members as well as relevant others that may be observed in advertising. From our study of social influences, we know that certain people are more likely to be imitated than others—e.g. those that are more similar to ourselves based on relevant factors such as age, social status, or ethnic group. Consider, for example, the poor man who is rejected by women because of his dandruff until he gets "with it" and uses Head 'n' Shoulders shampoo. Other dandruff sufferers are likely to learn from the model's experience. Generally, observations are made of overt behaviour, but some room is made for individual reasoning in learning from others. This perspective is clearly more realistic than that of the "Hard Core" view, but it should be noted that the strength of learning tends to be greater for that gained from own experience.

The *Cognitive* approach emphasises consumer *thinking* rather than mere behaviour—we will encounter this to a great extent when we study decision-making and attitudes. Here, the emphasis is on how people reason themselves to the consequences of their behaviour. Note that it is often somewhat more difficult to attempt to "get into" a consumer's head than it is to merely observe his or her behaviour, and what we "observe" is somewhat more subjective. Note also that a wealth of different factors influence people's thinking, and some expectations and assumptions that we hold tend to be culturally influenced (e.g., an Indian assumes that hard work will tend to lead to a promotion, while members of certain other cultures believe that personal relationships, and perhaps even luck, tend to be more important).

- **The *Biological* Approach Suggests** that most behaviour is determined by genetics or other biological bases. By this perspective, it is suggested that consumers eat the foods they eat in large part because the body craves these foods. Note that although craving for fatty foods seems quite maladaptive in today's society, it could have been very adaptive earlier in human history where food was scarce and obtaining as many calories as possible helped ensure survival. Clearly, this perspective is very misleading when one takes it as the *only* explanation of behaviour—for example, people in different cultures learn to enjoy various kinds of foods. The main implication of *biological determinism* is that the marketer must *adapt*—for example, food advertisements are more likely to be effective when people are hungry, and thus they might better be run in the late afternoon rather than in the late morning.
- **The Rational Expectations Perspective** is based on an economic way of looking at the World. Economists *assume* that people think rationally and have perfect information, even though they know very well that these assumptions are often unrealistic. However, despite the unrealistic assumptions made, economists often make relatively accurate predictions of human behaviour. (The Cognitive perspective, however, is able to identify certain significant exceptions to rational behaviour, however).
- **The *Psychoanalytic* Perspective** is based on the work of historical Maslow's Hierarchy of Needs. The late Abraham Maslow suggested the intuitively appealing notion that humans must satisfy the most basic objectives before they can move onto "higher level" ones. Thus, an individual must satisfy physiological needs (such as food and liquid) before he or she will be able to expend energy on less fundamental objectives such as safety. Only when basic objectives have been met will a person move on to seek such objectives as love and belonging, and only a small minority of people

make it as far as seeking self-actualisation.

Maslow's Hierarchy is useful in understanding different needs of consumers across the World. However, one must be careful not to take it too literally, since people may occasionally "swing" between needs. For example, a homeless person who currently does not have shelter may seek that out even though he or she is hungry.

Properties of Motivation. Motivation is described through several properties:

- *Motivation is composed of energy and direction.* A person may or may not have enough motivation to engage in a given activity. For example, a person may be motivated enough to go and shop for food, but not enough to engage in a comprehensive exercise programme.
- *Motives may be overt, hidden, and multiple*. Some motivations are publicly expressed (e.g., the desire to buy an energy efficient house), while others (e.g., the desire to look wealthy by buying a fancy car) are not. Individuals may also hold multiple motivations (e.g., buy a car *and* save money for retirement) which may conflict.
- *Many motivations are driven by the desire for tension reduction* (e.g., eliminate thirst or hunger).
- *Motivations can be driven by both internal and external factors*. That is, a person may want a painting either because he or she likes it (internal motivation) or because this will give her status among the artistic elite (external).
- *Motivations may have either a positive or negative valence*—people may either be motivated to achieve something (e.g., get a promotion at work) or avoid something (e.g., being hospitalised without having adequate insurance).
- *Consumers are motivated to achieve goals.* Achieving these goals may require sustained activity over time (e.g., exercising every day for months or years) as opposed to just taking some action once.
- *Consumers maintain a balance between the desires for stability and variety*. Most consumers want some variety (e.g., they do not want to eat the same meal every day), but also want a certain stability (they do not want to try an entirely new food every day).
- *Motivation reflects individual differences*. Different consumers

are motivated to achieve different things, and it may be difficult to infer motivations from looking at actual behaviour without understanding these differences in desired outcomes.

The reality that consumers are frequently motivated by multiple motives suggests a possibility that motives may conflict. Three main types of conflict exists:

- *Approach-avoidance.* One alternative has both positive consequences (that one wishes to seek out) and negative consequences (that one wants to avoid). For example, eating a large banana split is an enjoyable experience ("approach"), but is contains a lot of calories ("avoidance") and may make one feel ill later (another avoidance).
- *Approach-approach.* A consumer wants to do two incompatible things at the same time. A classic example is "Rainman's" desire both to stay with his brother and stay at the institution. Another example is a consumer who only has one week's vacation but wants equally to go to Hawaii and Greenland, but has time and money only for one of the two.
- *Avoidance-avoidance.* A consumer does not want to go for either of two alternatives, but must choose the lesser of two evils. For example, the consumer does not want to pay for car insurance, but does not want to get into an accident or get caught by the police without it. A "work ethic disadvantaged" student does not want to study, but does not want to fail his or her courses, either.

The Means-End Chain : Consumers often buy products not because of their attributes *per se* but rather because of the ultimate benefits that these attributes provide, in turn leading to the satisfaction of ultimate values. For example, a consumer may not be particularly interested in the chemistry of plastic roses, but might reason as follows:

Highly reliable synthetic content of roses →

Roses will stay in original condition for a long time →

Significant other will appreciate the roses longer →

Significant other will continue to love one → Self esteem.

The important thing in a means-end chain is to start with an *attribute*, a concrete characteristic of the product, and then logically progress to a series of consequences (which tend to become progressively more abstract) that end with a *value* being satisfied. Thus, each chain *must start with an attribute and end with a value.*

An important implication of means-end chains is that it is usually most effective in advertising to *focus on higher-level items*. For example, in the flower example above, an individual giving the flowers to the significant other might better be portrayed than the flowers alone.

Personality and Consumer Behaviour. Traditional research in marketing has not been particularly successful in finding a link between personality and consumer behaviour. Part of the problem here is that much of the theory has been developed by clinical psychologists who have tended to work with maladjusted people. Not surprisingly, research that sought to predict, based on standard personality inventories, which kinds of consumers would buy Coverlets as opposed to Fords was not successful.

Emotion. Emotion impacts marketing efforts in several ways. One purpose is to get *attention* to a stimulus (since emotionally charged individuals tend to be less predictable than calmer ones, there has been an evolutionary advantage in paying attention to emotion). Secondly, emotion influences *information processing*. In general, happy people tend to scrutinise arguments given (e.g., purported benefits of using a product) somewhat less, since they do not want to lose their happy moods by doing too much thinking. In general, happy ads are somewhat better *liked*, and may be better *remembered*. *Empathy* may also increase liking for the ad and the sponsoring product.

Attitudes

Definition. Consumer attitudes are a composite of a consumer's (1) beliefs about, (2) feelings about, (3) and behavioural intentions toward some object—within the context of marketing, usually a brand or retail store. These components are viewed together since they are highly interdependent and together represent forces that influence how the consumer will react to the object.[16]

Beliefs. The first component is *beliefs*. A consumer may hold both positive beliefs toward an object (e.g., coffee tastes good) as well as negative beliefs (e.g., coffee is easily spilled and stains papers). In addition, some beliefs may be neutral (coffee is black), and some may be differ in valance depending on the person or the situation (e.g., coffee is hot and stimulates—good on a cold morning, but not good on a hot summer evening when one wants to sleep). Note also that the beliefs that consumer's hold need not be accurate (e.g., that pork contains little fat), and some beliefs may, upon closer examination, be contradictory (e.g., that a historical figure was a good person but also owned slaves).

Since a consumer holds many beliefs, it may often be difficult to get down to a "bottom line" overall belief about whether an object such as McDonald's is overall good or bad. The Multiattribute (also sometimes known as the Fishbein) Model attempts to summarise overall attitudes into one score using the equation:

That is, for each belief, we take the weight, or importance (W_i) of that belief and multiply it with its evaluation (X_{ib}). For example, a consumer believes that the taste of a beverage is moderately important, or a 4 on a scale from 1 to 7. He or she believes that coffee tastes very good, or a 6 on a scale from 1 to 7. Thus, the product here is 4(6)=24. On the other hand, he or she believes that the potential of a drink to stain is extremely important (7), and coffee fares moderately badly, at a score -4, on this attribute (since this is a negative belief, we now take negative numbers from -1 to -7, with -7 being worst). Thus, we now have 7(–4)=–28. Had these two beliefs been the only beliefs the consumer held, his or her total, or aggregated, attitude would have been 24+(–28)=–4. In practice, of course, consumers tend to have many more beliefs that must each be added to obtain an accurate measurement.

Affect. Consumers also hold certain feelings toward brands or other objects. Sometimes these feelings are based on the beliefs (e.g., a person feels nauseated when thinking about a hamburger because of the tremendous amount of fat it contains), but there may also be feelings, which are relatively independent of beliefs. For example, an extreme environmentalist may believe that cutting down trees is morally wrong, but may have positive affect toward Christmas trees because he or she unconsciously associates these trees with the experience that he or she had at Christmas as a child.

Behavioural Intention. The behavioural intention is what the consumer plans to do with respect to the object (e.g., buy or not buy the brand). As with affect, this is sometimes a logical consequence of beliefs (or affect), but May sometimes reflect other circumstances—e.g. although a consumer does not really like a restaurant, he or she will go there because it is a hangout for his or her friends.

Attitude-Behaviour Consistency. Consumers often do not behave consistently with their attitudes for several reasons:

- *Ability.* He or she may be unable to do so. Although junior high school student likes pick-up trucks and would like to buy one, she may lack a driver's license.
- *Competing demands for resources.* Although the above student

would like to buy a pickup truck on her sixteenth birthday, she would rather have a computer, and has money for only one of the two.

- *Social influence.* A student thinks that smoking is really cool, but since his friends think it's disgusting, he does not smoke.
- *Measurement problems.* Measuring attitudes is difficult. In many situations, consumers do not consciously set out to enumerate how positively or negatively they feel about mopeds, and when a market researcher asks them about their beliefs about mopeds, how important these beliefs are, and their evaluation of the performance of mopeds with respect to these beliefs, consumers often do not give very reliable answers. Thus, the consumers may act consistently with their true attitudes, which were never uncovered because an erroneous measurement was made.

Attitude Change Strategies. Changing attitudes is generally *very difficult*, particularly when consumers suspect that the marketer has a self-serving agenda in bringing about this change (e.g., to get the consumer to buy more or to switch brands).

Changing affect. One approach is to try to change affect, which may or may not involve getting consumers to change their beliefs. One strategy uses the approach of *classical conditioning* try to "pair" the product with a liked stimulus. For example, we "pair" a car with a beautiful woman. Alternatively, we can try to get people to like the advertisement and hope that this liking will "spill over" into the purchase of a product. For example, the Pillsbury Doughboy does not really emphasise the conveyance of much information to the consumer; instead, it attempts to create a warm, fuzzy image. Although Energizer Bunny ads try to get people to believe that their batteries last longer, the main emphasis is on the likeable bunny. Finally, products which are better known, through the *mere exposure* effect, tend to be better liked—that is, the more a product is advertised and seen in stores, the more it will generally be liked, *even if consumers to do not develop any specific beliefs about the product*.[17]

Changing behaviour. People like to believe that their behaviour is rational; thus, once they use our products, chances are that they will continue unless someone is able to get them to switch. One way to get people to switch to our brand is to use temporary price discounts and coupons; however, when consumers buy a product on deal, they may justify the purchase based on that deal (i.e., the low price) and may then switch to other brands on deal later. A better way to get people to switch to our brand is to at least temporarily obtain better shelf space so that the product is more convenient. Consumers are less likely to use this availability as a rationale for their purchase and may continue to buy the product even when the product is less conveniently located. (Notice, by the way, that this represents a case of shaping).

Changing beliefs. Although attempting to change beliefs is the obvious way to attempt attitude change, particularly when consumers hold unfavorable or inaccurate ones, this is often difficult to achieve because consumers tend to resist. Several approaches to belief change exist:

- *Change currently held beliefs.* It is generally very difficult to attempt to change beliefs that people hold, particularly those that are strongly held, *even if they are inaccurate*. For example, the petroleum industry advertised for a long time that its profits were lower than were commonly believed, and provided extensive factual evidence in its advertising to support this reality. Consumers were suspicious and rejected this information, however.
- *Change the importance of beliefs.* Although the sugar manufacturers would undoubtedly like to decrease the importance of healthy teeth, it is usually not feasible to make beliefs less important—consumers are likely to reason, why, then, would you bother bringing them up in the first place? However, it may be possible to strengthen beliefs that favour us—e.g. a vitamin supplement manufacturer may advertise that it is extremely important for women to replace iron lost through menstruation. Most consumers already agree with this, but the belief can be made stronger.
- *Change ideal.* It usually difficult, and very risky, to attempt to change ideals, and only few firms succeed. For example, Hard Candy may have attempted to change the ideal away from traditional beauty toward more unique self-expression.

One-sided vs. Two-sided appeals. Attitude research has shown that consumers often tend to react more favorably to advertisements which either (1) admit something negative about the sponsoring brand (e.g., the Volva is a clumsy Bus, but very safe) or (2) admits something positive about a competing brand (e.g., a competing supermarket has slightly lower prices, but offers less service and selection). Two-sided appeals must, contain overriding arguments why the sponsoring brand is ultimately superior—that is, in the above examples, the "but" part must be emphasised.

The Elaboration Likelihood Model (ELM) and Celebrity Endorsements. The ELM suggests that consumers will scrutinise claims more in important situations than in unimportant ones. For example, we found that in the study of people trying to get ahead of others in a line to use photocopiers, the compliance rate was about fifty per cent when people just asked to get ahead. However, when the justification "... because I have to make copies" was added, compliance increased to 80 per cent. Since the reason offered really did not add substantive information, we conclude that it was not extensively analysed—in the jargon of the theory, "elaboration" was low.

The ELM suggests that for "unimportant" products, elaboration will be low. For example, a basket ball player is likely to be effective in endorsing athletic shoes, but not in endorsing automobiles. On the other hand, a nationally syndicated auto columnist would be successful in endorsing cars, but not athletic shoes. All of them, however, could endorse fast food restaurants effectively.[18]

Appeal approaches. Several approaches to appeal may be used. The use of *affect* to induce *empathy* with advertising characters may increase attraction to a product, but may backfire if consumers believe that people's feelings are being exploited. *Fear appeals* appear to work only if (1) an optimal level of fear is evoked—not so much that people tune it out, but enough to scare people into action *and* (2) a way to avoid the feared stimulus is explicitly indicated—e.g. gingivitis and tooth loss can be avoided by using this mouth wash. *Humor* appears to be effective in gaining attention, but does not appear to increase persuasion in practice. In addition, a more favorable attitude toward the advertisement may be created by humorous advertising, which may in turn result in increased sales. *Comparative advertising*, which is illegal in many countries, often increases sales for the sponsoring brand, but may backfire in certain cultures.

Self-Concept, Situational Influences and Life-style

The self-concept. The consumer faces several possible selves. The *actual* self reflects how the individual actually is, although the consumer may not be aware of that reality (e.g., many anorexia consumers who are dangerously thin believe that they are in fact fat). In contrast, the *ideal* self reflects a self that a person would like to have, but does not in fact have. For example, a couch potato may want to be a World famous athlete, but may have no actual athletic ability. The *private* self is one that is not intentionally exposed to others. For example, a police officer may like and listen to remix music in private, but project a *public* self-image of a country music enthusiast, playing country songs at work where police officers are portrayed as heroes. The key here is to keep in mind which kind of self we are trying to reach in promotional messages. If we appeal to the hidden self, for example, we must be careful to make our appeals subtle and hint, if appropriate, on how the individual's confidentiality and privacy can be enhanced.[19]

Individuals will often seek to augment and enhance their self-concepts, and it may be possible to market products that help achieve this goal.

Life-styles. Self-concept often translates into a person's life-styles, or the way that he or she lives his or her life. For example, a person may be very materialistic, preferring to wear flashy clothes and drive expensive cars, or prefer instead a simpler life with fewer visible status symbols. Attempts have been made to classify consumers into various segments based on their life-styles public recognition, but only the Achievers have the resources to bring this about. A global analogue is the Global Scan.

Situational influences. Specific circumstances often influence consumer behaviour. For example, consumers in a rush are likely to take the most convenient product available. Consumers whose attention is demanded elsewhere are likely to disregard commercial messages. Consumers shopping for a special occasion (e.g., a wedding) may buy different products.

Consumer Decision Making

Definitions. Consumer decision-making comes about as an attempt to solve consumer problems. A *problem* refers to "a discrepancy between a desired state and an ideal state which is sufficient to arouse and activate a decision process." Thus, problems can be major (e.g., a consumer has been fired and is without a job) or minor (e.g., the consumer lacks an eraser necessary to take an exam the next day), and the broader and more ambiguous a problem is, the more potential solutions are generally available (see class slides for examples).

Consumer Problem Recognition. Consumers often note problems by comparing their current, or actual, situation, explicitly or implicitly, to some desired situation. In terms of the "big picture," what is compared may be the totality of one's life-style. Once a discrepancy is found, a determination is found as to whether this is large enough to warrant action, in which case a search for solutions is initiated.

Problems come in several different types. A problem may be an *active* one (e.g., you have a headache and would like as quick a solution as possible) or *inactive*— you are not aware that your situation is a problem (e.g., a consumer is not aware that he or she could have more energy with a new vitamin). Problems may be *acknowledged* (e.g., a consumer is aware that his or her car does not accelerate well enough or *unacknowledged* (e.g., a consumer will not acknowledge that he or she consumes too much alcohol). Finally, needs can be relatively specific (generic), as in the need for enjoyment (which can be satisfied many different ways), or specific, as in the need for professional attire to wear at a new job.

Creating problems for consumers is a way to increase sales, albeit a questionably ethical one. One way to create new problems, and resultant needs, is to create a new ideal state. It may also be possible to create dissatisfaction with current states—e.g., a firm may publicise current crime statistics to increase the sales of handguns and alarms. Many vocational training schools advertise that better careers than the consumer's current one are available upon graduation (a promise on which, by the way, they may not deliver in the end).

Consumers often do not consider all alternatives. Some are not known (the "unawareness" set), some were once known but are not readily accessible in memory (the "inert" set), others are ruled out as unsatisfactory (the "inept" set—e.g., Glad bags attempts to get "bargain bags" into that set), and those that are considered represent the "evoked" set, from which one alternative is likely to be purchased.

The amount of effort a consumer puts into searching depends on a number of factors such as the market (how many competitors are there, and how great are differences between brands expected to be?), product characteristics (how important is this product? How complex is the product? How obvious are indications of quality?), consumer characteristics (how interested is a consumer, generally, in analysing product characteristics and making the best possible deal?), and situational characteristics (as previously discussed).

Two interesting issues in decisions are *variety seeking* (where consumers seek to try new brands not because these brands are expected to be "better" in any way, but rather because the consumer wants a "change of pace," and *"impulse" purchases*.

Consumer Outlet Selection[20]

Retail evolution and consumer choice. For many products, consumers frequently have numerous choices as to *where* they are going to actually obtain the product. Although we are used to thinking of buying automobiles only from dealership, for example, it is today possible to buy them through brokers or fleet sales organisations that may both (1) offer a lower price and/or (2) provide the help of a neutral third party which does not have a vested interest in the sales of one make over the other.

In general, the evolution of diversity in the retail scene has provided consumers with more choice. In the old days, most consumers had access only to "general" stores for most products. Gradually, in urban environments, specialty and discount stores evolved. Today, a consumer may generally choose to buy most products either at a relatively high price, frequently with a significant amount of service, in a specialty store, or with lower service in a discount store. A special case of the discount store is the *category killer*—a store that tends to specialise in some limited area (e.g., electronics), lacking the breadth of a traditional discount store often undercutting the traditional discount store on price (which they are able to do because of the bargaining power that results from high buying volumes of a narrow assortment of merchandise from the same manufacturer).

"At home" shopping and electronic commerce. During the last several decades, the incidence of "at home" shopping has increased. The growth of catalog sales can be traced to advances in computer technology and subsequent list availability (as we discussed in the section of direct marketing segmentation methods). A more recent development is Internet based marketing. Although sales are modest in this domain at the moment, it is too early to judge the total potential of this medium. Although many of the concerns that consumers hold about computer crime tend to be exaggerated and/or largely unwarranted, public fears are a major holdback. Another problem is the demographics of computer and Internet use—the majority of Indian consumers, and certainly the great majority of residents of even highly industrialised countries, are not regular Internet users. Certain products specifically aimed at heavy Internet users (e.g., records, software) and products/

services that require a high level of customisation (e.g., airline tickets) may find good opportunities. An interesting problem with Internet commerce, which may well have spillover effects outside the realm of the Net, is the relative ease with which consumers may compare prices of different retailers, resulting in intense price competition.

Store positioning. Positioning of retail stores is essential. In general, stores, which *excel on a significant dimension,* seem to perform better—for example, Nordstrom's excels through its intense customer service, while Wal-Mart excels through its efficiency and low prices. (In a course on marketing strategy or retailing, you will probably discuss the issue of the importance of *balanced markets*—it is healthier if different firms have different strategies, so that everyone will not be competing intensely on the same variables). Stores which fall somewhere in between—e.g., Sears—tend to do less well since they get "stuck in the middle" and have to compete against both. Obviously, there is a limit to how strongly you can move toward one extreme. For example, if Nordstrom were to double its prices and even double its service, that position would be untenable, and certain extreme discount stores that offer lower prices than Wal-Mart tend not to be successful because they are ultimately not satisfactory to consumers.

Public Policy Issues[21]

Throughout the term, we have considered marketing practices, which may harm consumers. Two main issues are (1) deceptive marketing practices (such as misleading advertising) and (2) the marketing of dangerous or otherwise harmful products (e.g., tobacco). The following are some ethical problems that occur in marketing, and the question arises as to which, if any, kind of government intervention is appropriate:

- *Marketing efforts may encourage excess consumption* (e.g., products that consumers cannot afford and do not really need). Note, however, that there are many gray areas—e.g. cosmetics, video games, and even something as politically correct as a gourmet coffee houses. A special case involves marketing to children, whose parents may be coerced, often out of guilt, to buy questionable items aimed at children.
- *Deceptive marketing practices*: Products claim benefits which really do not result from use of the product (as is done by numerous manufacturers of nutritional supplements); advertising may be misleading (may not indicate the true

cost of a product up front or may contain "fine print" that the consumer is unlikely to see or understand).

- *Products are unhealthy* (e.g., many children's foods contain excessive fat).

Government action is often considered, although it may not always be effective. For example, although the government requires the use of warning labels on some products, manufacturers will often try to "water down" the warnings as much as possible. Further, the prevalence of warning labels today may desensitise consumers since reading all of them carefully would provide the consumer with information overload.[22]

Consumer protection entails protecting the rights and interests of the consumers in matters of availability, quality, quantity and price of goods and services. It infect promotes the concept of value for money and enhances the trust between the customer and the producer or provider. Consumer Protection policy recognises that consumers often face imbalances in economic terms, educational levels and bargaining power and that the consumers should have the right of access to non-hazardous products as well as the right to promote just, equitable and sustainable economic and social development.

Consumers are now participate in a global market, and at the mercy of the market forces. In a large country like India the ills of globalisation and liberalisation are visible as a result both the consumers and law – market are equally worried. A net of legal protections provided have proved to be inadequate to protect the consumer from exolitation. Globalisation is gaining strength all around us and we need to reinforce and strengthen our system to meet its challenges. There is a need to ensure that India does not become a dumping ground for sub-standard products. Consumer protection as a move consumer movement has yet to take off in the real sense. There are laws can only protect the consumers protecting the consumer. Moreover law can only protect the consumers through rules. Which are essentially national and which can only be enforced within national boundaries.

Consumers are now seeking protection through legislations that have a global reach because the general laws and market forces have proved to be inadequate to protect them. Many consumer protection laws either relate to the terms and conditions of contracts that consumers make with suppliers for the supply of goods and services, or intended to encourage the making of such contracts (marketing, packaging and provision of information). Since

1960 most developed countries with common legal system, and most recently countries of Asia have enacted significant consumer protection legislations. However such laws are national and operate only within the geographical limits of the enacting jurisdiction.

Consumerism is a process through which the consumers seeks, redress, restitution and remedy for their dissatisfaction and frustration with the help of their organised and unorganised efforts and activities. It is in fact a social movement seeking to protect the rights of the consumers in relation to the producers and providers of services.

In its wider perspective it in is an the agenda of administrative reforms for greater accountability, responsiveness and transparency through the technique of decentralisation, debureaucratisation and devolved planning process. It's a part of the ongoing debate for good governance which recognises the right to information as a prerequisite. In many of the developed countries consumerism has over the time developed into a sound force designed to aid and protect the consumer by exerting legal, moral and economic pressure on producers and providers of services.

The objectives of the guidelines for consumer protection are :

(1) To assist countries in achieving or maintaining adequate protection for their populations as consumer.

(2) To facilitate production and distribution patterns responsive to the needs and desires of consumers.

(3) To encourage high level of ethical conduct for those engaged in the production and distribution of goods and services to consumer group.

(4) To assist countries in curbing abusive business practices by all enterprises at the national and international levels which adversely affect consumer.

(5) To facilitate the development of independent consumer group.

(6) To encourage the development of market conditions which provide consumers with greater choice at lower prices.

The guidelines put enormous responsibility on the government to protect the consumers. It states that the Govt. should develop, strengthen or maintain a strong consumer protection policy, taking into account the guidelines set out. For doing so each Govt must set its own priorities for the protection of consumers in accordance with the economic and social circumstances of the country, and the needs of its population, and bearing needs that the guidelines are intended to meet are following:

(a) The protection of consumers from hazards to their health and safety;

(b) The promotion and protection of the economic interests of consumers;

(c) The access of consumers to adequate information to enable them to make informed choices according to individual wishes and needs;

(d) Consumer Education;

(e) Availability of effective consumers redress;

(f) Freedom to form consumer and other relevant groups or organisations and the opportunity of such organisations to present their view in decision- making processes affecting them.

The Govt. should also provide or maintain adequate infrastructure to develop, implement and monitor consumer protection policies. Special care should be taken to ensure that measures for consumer protection are implemented for the benefit of all sections of the population particularly the rural population. Apart from these the guidelines also provide that Govt should establish or maintain legal or administrative measures to enable consumers or, as appropriate, relevant organisations to obtain redress through formal or informal procedures to take particular account of the needs of low–income consumer.

Consumer Protection in India

Even though the consumer movement as such is a new phenomenon in India, yet the concept is quite old, Mahatma Gandhi attached great importance to what he described as the poor consumer, who according to him should be the principal beneficiary of the consumer movement. He said, "a consumer is most important visitor on our premises. He is not an interruption to our work, he is the purpose of it. We are not doing a favour to a consumer by giving him an opportunity. He is doing us a favour by giving us an opportunity to serve him". However, inspite of these views of the father of the nation, consumerism as a moment is still in its infancy in our country, but of late it is gaining momentum.

In the recent past the Govt has accorded a high priority to the issues of consumer protection and has initiated other steps to promote a responsible and responsive consumer movement in the country.[21]

Consumer Protection; Legal Framework

In India various legislations, intended to protect the consumer against different forms of exploitatuin have been enacted. The important ones being drugs control act 1950, Indian standards Institution At 1952, Prevention of Food Adulteration Act 1958, Standards of weight and measures Act 1985 etc. However, these Acts were mainly punitive and preventive in nature, therefore, the consumer did not have any effective mechanism or institutional arrangement for the speedy redressal of their grievances. Keeping in view the UN guidelines and in order to plug a number of loopholes in various legislations, the govt enacted the consumer Protection Act in 1968. It was an Act to provide for the better protection of the interest of consumers and for that purpose for the establishment of consumer disputes.

The Consumer Protection Act, 1986

The Consumer Protection Act of 1986 was a Milestone in the consumer protection movement in the country. It has been enacted with a view to provide speedy and in–expensive remedy to consumer aims at protecting the consumers from exploitation by traders and service providers. The Act prescribes the establishment of consumer redressal agencies. It provides that the state Govt. shall establish a consumer dispute redressal forum known as district forum for each district and consumer disputes redressal Commission shall also be established. The national commission will be headed by a President, who shall be a sitting or retired Judge of the Supreme Court and shall consist of four other members, one of whom shall be a sitting or retired Judge of High Court and shall consist of two members one of whom shall be a woman. Similarly, the District forum shall consist of a President who shall be a sitting or retired Judge of supreme court and shall consist of four other members, one of the whom shall be woman. The state commission will consist of a president, who shall be setting or retired Judge of High Court and shall consist of two members one of whom shall be a woman. Similarly, the district forum shall consist of a President who shall be a sitting or retired District judge or qualified to be a district judge. The District Forum shall consist of two other members, one of whom shall be a woman.

Central Consumer Protection Council

The Act provides that the Central Govt may, be notification establish a council to be known as the Central Consumer Protection Council.

The Council shall consist of the following members, namely :

(a) The Minister in charge of Consumer Affairs in the Central Govt. who shall be its Chairman and (b) Such number of other official or non-official members representing such interest as may be prescribed. The Central Council shall meet as and when necessary but at least one meeting of the council shall be held every year. The objectives of the Central Council shall be to promote and protect the right of the consumer such as :

(i) The Right to be protected against the marketing of goods and services which are hours to life and property.

(ii) The right to be informed bout the utility, quantity, potenty, purity, standard and price of goods and services as the case may be so as to protect the consumer against unfair trade practices.

(iii) The right to be assured, wherever possible, access to variety of goods and services at competitive prices.

(iv) The right to be heard and to be assured that consumers interests will receive due consideration at appropriate forums.

(v) The right to such redressal against unfair trade practices or restrictive trade practices or unscrupulous exploitation of consumers.

(vi) The right to consumer education.

Similarly, the state Govt. may establish the state Consumer Protection Council. The state Council shall consist of the following members; namely

(a) The minister in-charge of Consumer Affairs in the state Govt who shall be its Chairman.

(b) Such number of other official or non official members representing such interests as may be prescribed by the state Govt. The state Council shall meet as and when necessary but not less than two meeting shall be held every year. The objects of the state Council shall be to promote and protect within the state, the rights of the consumers.

The Consumer Protection (Amendment) Act 2000 provides for the setting up of the District Consumer Protection Council. The state Govt. shall establish for every district by notification a council to be known as the District Consumer Protection Council. The District Consumer Protection Council shall consist of the collector of the district, who shall be its chairman. The state Govt. may prescribe such number of other official and non official member representing such interests. The District Council shall be to promote and protect within the district the right of the consumers as laid down in clauses (a) to (f) of section 6.23

It also define the procedure of making complaints which shall made under Section 12 (1). According to this section a complaint in relation to any goods sold or delivered or agreed to be sold or delivered or any services provided or agreed to be provided may be filed with the District Forum by (a) the consumer to whom such good are sold or deliveredvered or agreed to be sold or delivered or such service provided or agreed to be provided; (be any recognised consumer association where the consumer to whom the goods sold or delivered or agreed to be sold or delivered or service provided or agreed to be provided is a member of such association or not; (c) one or more consumer, where there are numerous consumers having the same interests, with the permission of the District Forum, on behalf of, or for the benefit of all consumers so interested; or (d) the central Govt. or the state Govt, as the case may be, either in its individual capacity or as a representative of Interest of the consumer in general.

IT further provides that every complaint filed district Fermentor sub-section (1) Shall be accompanied with such amount of fee and payable in such manner as may be prescribed. On receipt of a complaint the District Forum may by order allow the complaint to be proceeded.

References

1. American Marketing Association (1960), *Marketing Definitions : A Glossary of Marketing Terms*, Chicago : AMA.
2. ASSOCHAM (1990), *Consumer Awareness : Initiatives from Government, Industry and Consumer Organisaitons,* New Delhi : ASSOCHAM.
3. ASSOCHAM (1994), *Spurious and Counterfeit Products - How to Combat the Menance*? Souvenir by ASOCHAM on World Consumer Rights Day, New Delhi : ASSOCHAM.
4. Bellur, Venkatakrishna V., and Harold W. Berkman (1987), *Readings in Marketing Management*, Bombay : Himalaya Publishing House.
5. Kotler, Philip (1994), *Marketing Management : Analysis, Planning, Implementation and Control*, New Delhi : Prentice Hall of India.
6. Krishnamurthi, S. (1988), *Guide to Economic Legislation*, Allahabad: Orient Law House.
7. Michael R. Solman, *Consumer Behaviour,* published in Person Education, India, 2002.

8. *Indian Marketing : The Case Studies,* New Delhi : Anmol Publications, 1991.

9. Kotler, Philip (1994), *Marketing Management : Analysis, Planning, Implementation, and Control*, New Delhi : Prentice Hall of India.

10. Krishnamurthi, S. (1988), *Guide to Economic Legislation,* Allahabad: Orient Law House.

11. Based on Laurie Freeman, "FDA Snaps at Oral-Care Ads," Advertising Age, October 10, 1988, pp. 3, 76, and Laurie Freeman, "Colgate, FDA Battle Over Plaque," *Advertising Age*, April 23, 1990, p. 20.

12. Based on John Tierney, "With 'Social marketing,' Condoms Combat AIDS," The New York Times, September 18, 1990, pp. A1, A10.

13. "Greener Pastures," *American Demographics*, April 1991, p. 12.

14. Jac Goldstucker, "The influence of Culture on Channels of Distribution," in Robert L. King (ed), *Marketing and the New Science of Planning, American Marketing Association*, Chicago, 1968, p. 470.'

15. Russel I. Haley, "Benefit Segmentation-20 Years Later," *Journal of Consumer Marketing,* 1:6 No. 2, 1984.

16. Jan-Benedict E.M. Steenkamp, frenkel ter Hofstede, and Michale Wedel, "A Cross - National Investigation into the Individual and National Cultural Antecedents of Consumer Invectiveness", *Journal of Marketing,* 63, No. 7 (1999), pp. 55-69.

17. Melanie wallendorf, "The Formation of Aesthetic Criteria through Social Structure and Social Institution", in Jerry C. Olson, ed; Advances in Consumer Research 7, Ann Arbor, MI: Association for Consumer Research, 1980, pp. 3-6.

18. Richard T. LaPiere, *Sociology*, McGraw-Hill, New York, 1946.

19. Henry, *Cultural Values*, pp. 121-27.

20. Michael Quinn, "Don't Aim That Pack At Us," *Time*, January 29, 1990, p. 60.

21. C.K. Prahalad and Venkatram Ramaswamy, "Co-opting Customer Competence, "Harvard Business Review (January-Feb. 2000): 79-87. Eric von Hipple, "Users as Innovators, "Technology Review 80 (Jan.-Feb.): 3-11; Jakki Mohr, Marketing of High-technology Products and services, Upper Saddle River, NJ : Prentic Hall 2001.

Index

Y